SURGICAL FINALS

Structured Answer and Essay Questions

Second Edition

Ramanathan Visvanathan BM FRCS
Consultant Surgeon, Bronglais General Hospital, Aberystwyth, Honorary Lecturer, University of Wales College of Medicine, Surgical Tutor, Royal College of Surgeons of England, Lately Honorary Senior Lecturer and Assistant Director, Professorial Surgical Unit, St Bartholomew's Hospital, London

John S P Lumley MS FRCS
Professor of Surgery, St Bartholomew's and the Royal London School of Medicine and Dentistry and Honorary Consultant Surgeon St Bartholomew's Hospital, London, Member of Council, Royal College of Surgeons of England, Past World President International College of Surgeons

PASTEST
Dedicated to your success

Knutsford
Cheshire
Telephone: 01565 752000

First edition 1997
Reprinted 1998
Second edition 1999
Reprinted 2001

ISBN: 0 906896 43 X

A catalogue record for this book is available from the British Library.

Typeset by **EDITEXT**, Charlesworth, Derbyshire.
Printed and bound in Great Britain by MPG Books Ltd, Bodmin, Cornwall

CONTENTS

Dedication

In memory of our fathers

PREFACE

With the current trend away from traditional essay questions for determining clinical knowledge, more and more examining bodies are introducing structured answer questions (SAQs) into undergraduate and postgraduate medical examinations. SAQs are designed to test problem-solving and decision-making in a structured and objective fashion, and are proving a reliable means of assessing knowledge and understanding in clinical practice. Many examiners also appreciate the fact that SAQs can be marked more quickly, more easily and often more accurately than essays. This book is intended for undergraduates preparing for their finals and for basic surgical trainees preparing for the MRCS/AFRCS examinations.

Section I consists of SAQs based on surgical knowledge in general. The reader is encouraged to write his or her answers in the boxes provided so that marks can be accurately allocated.

Section II contains model answers and marking schedules for every question. The authors have also included short comments to expand on each topic and to highlight common pitfalls that should be avoided.

Section III offers advice on how to approach essay questions with a selection of structured outlines on good essay planning and several genuine answers to a sample essay question complete with illuminating examiners' comments.

Section IV contains a selection of typical questions to provide invaluable essay writing practice.

The three appendices to the book contain additional material likely to be helpful to the reader. Appendix A is an analysis of the final examination in surgery which explains the evolution of assessment techniques and may also be useful to senior doctors who are involved with setting examinations.

Appendix B provides the reader with the opportunity to sit mock SAQ examination papers. Each paper provides an authentic mixture of examination topics. Appendix C groups the essay questions in Section IV into mock exam papers.

The book provides a range of questions to be used as a broad base for revision purposes. It may be used as a learning aid, together with surgical texts and other information sources, and it is also a valuable method of self-assessment enabling the reader to check his or her progress at each stage of the surgical course.

Acknowledgement

We wish to thank Yvonne Mallett for typing the drafts of the text.

REVISION CHECKLIST

Use this checklist to record your revision progress. Tick the subjects when you feel confident that you have covered them adequately. This will ensure that you do not forget to revise any key topics.

Chapter 1: Surgical Physiology

- ☐ Fluid and electrolyte therapy
- ☐ Acid-base balance
- ☐ Enteral and parenteral feeding
- ☐ Transfusion reactions

Chapter 2: Trauma and Burns

- ☐ ATLS
- ☐ Head injury assessment
- ☐ Cervical spine injury
- ☐ Thoracic injury
- ☐ Blunt abdominal trauma
- ☐ Fracture of pelvis and long bones
- ☐ Assessment of burns
- ☐ Colloid and crystalloid therapy in burns

Chapter 3: Orthopaedics

- ☐ Osteoarthritis of the hip
- ☐ Rheumatoid arthritis
- ☐ Osteomyelitis
- ☐ Bone tumours
- ☐ Kyphoscoliosis

Chapter 4: Neurosurgery

- ☐ Head injury
- ☐ Meningomyelocoele
- ☐ Hydrocephalus
- ☐ Hypothalamic/pituitary lesions
- ☐ Peripheral nerve injuries

Chapter 5: Eyes, ENT and Skin

- ☐ The painful red eye
- ☐ Retinoblastoma
- ☐ Glaucoma
- ☐ Uveitis
- ☐ Nose bleed

- ☐ Chronic sinusitis
- ☐ Otitis media
- ☐ Tonsillitis
- ☐ Melanoma
- ☐ Squamous carcinoma
- ☐ Basal cell carcinoma

Chapter 6: Endocrinology, Breast and Chest Diseases

- ☐ Toxic goitre
- ☐ Thyroid malignancy
- ☐ Parathyroid hyperplasia
- ☐ Cervical adenopathy
- ☐ Adrenal tumours
- ☐ Benign breast disease
- ☐ Nipple discharge
- ☐ Breast cancer
- ☐ Lung cancer
- ☐ Lung abscess
- ☐ Coronary bypass surgery

Chapter 7: Upper Alimentary Tract

- ☐ Tongue lesions
- ☐ Salivary gland lesions
- ☐ Oesophageal stricture
- ☐ Peptic ulcer disease
- ☐ Gastric cancer
- ☐ Splenomegaly

Chapter 8: Liver, Gall Bladder and Pancreas

- ☐ Cirrhosis and portal hypertension
- ☐ Gall bladder: inflammation and stones
- ☐ Obstructive jaundice
- ☐ Pancreatitis

Chapter 9: Small and Large Bowel

- ☐ Bowel obstruction including hernia
- ☐ Appendicitis
- ☐ Ischaemic bowel
- ☐ Peritonitis

- ☐ Colonic polyps and cancer
- ☐ Inflammatory bowel disease
- ☐ Perianal lesions

Chapter 10: Urology

- ☐ Renal tumours and stones
- ☐ Bladder tumours and stones
- ☐ Urinary retention and incontinence
- ☐ Prostatic enlargement
- ☐ Testicular tumours
- ☐ Urethral stricture

Chapter 11: Vascular Surgery

- ☐ Carotid artery disease
- ☐ Cervical rib syndrome
- ☐ Aortic aneurysms
- ☐ Acute and chronic lower limb ischaemia
- ☐ Lower limb amputation
- ☐ Varicose veins
- ☐ Deep venous thrombosis

ABBREVIATIONS

ABG	Arterial blood gases estimation
ATLS	Advanced trauma life support systems
AXR	Abdominal X-ray (antero-posterior)
BP	Blood pressure
Ca^{++}	Calcium ions
CL^-	Chloride ions
CO_2	Carbon dioxide
CT	Computerised tomogram
CVP	Central venous pressure
CXR	Chest X-ray
ERCP	Endoscopic retrograde cholangio pancreatogram
ESR	Erythrocyte sedimentation rate
FBC	Full blood count
FNAC	Fine needle aspiration cytology
H^+	Protons or hydrogen ions
H_2O	Water
Hb	Haemoglobin
HCO_3^-	Bicarbonate ions
hr	Hour
ICP	Intra-cranial pressure
INR	International coagulation ratio
IV	Intravenous
IVU	Intravenous urography
K^+	Potassium ions
kcal	Kilocalorie
KCl	Potassium chloride
kg	Kilogram
Kpa	Kilopascals
l	Litre
LFT	Liver function test
ml	Millilitre
Mg^{++}	Magnesium ions
MRI	Magnetic resonance imaging
Na^+	Sodium ions
NaCl	Sodium chloride
O_2	Oxygen
OGD	Oesophago–gastro–duodenoscopy
PCV	Packed cell volume
PO_4^{---}	Phosphate ions
PTA	Percutaneous transluminal angioplasty
U&E	Urea and electrolytes
U/S	Ultrasound scan
WBC	White blood count

RECOMMENDED READING

General surgical texts

Clinical Examination of the Patient
Lumley JSP and Bouloux PMG, Butterworth Heinemann, 1994.
This book, with 486 colour photographs, serves as a useful guide for formulating and perfecting examination techniques.

Hamilton Bailey's Physical Signs
Demonstration of Physical Signs in Surgery
Lumley JSP (Ed.), 18th edition, Butterworth–Heinemann, 1997.
The recent edition of this well-known book on clinical diagnosis contains many new illustrations on the spectrum of surgical diseases and highlights the salient features of their diagnosis.

Lecture Notes in General Surgery
Ellis H and Calne R, 8th edition, Blackwell Scientific, 1992.
In this text, each surgical disease is classified with useful sections on pathology and management. This is especially helpful for learning how to write structured essay plans.

Demonstrations of Physical Signs: Picture Tests
JSP Lumley, S Chan, H Harris and MOM Zongana, Butterworth–Heinemann, 2000.

Essential Surgery: Problems, Diagnosis and Management
Burkitt HG, 2nd edition, Churchill Livingstone, 1995.
A popular textbook of general surgery aimed at clinical students. Its main advantages are its very readable style, clear explanations of the pathophysiological basis of surgical problems and illustrated synopses of the main stages of common surgical operations.

The Washington Manual of Surgery
Doherty GM et al., Little Brown & Co, 1997.
This book, which fits into the pocket of the white coat, provides the medical student, the house office and the surgical resident with a ready and easily accessible source of information on surgical diagnosis and treatment. It is written by surgical residents with input from house officers and is thus well-focused on the surgical knowledge base required by the newly qualified doctor.

Bailey and Love's New Short Practice of Surgery
Mann CV, Russell RCG and Williams NS, 22nd edition, Chapman & Hall, 1995.
A complete reference textbook that forms the basis of surgery after the Finals.

Orthopaedic texts

Essentials of Orthopaedic Examination
Hammer A, 3rd edition, Edward Arnold, 1994.
A small, clearly illustrated book which adopts a systematic approach to its examination schemes.

Physical Signs in Orthopaedics
Klenerman L and Walsh HJ, BMJ Publishing Group, 1994.
Over 200 black and white photographs with questions and answers. A useful revision aid for the clinicals.

Clinical Orthopaedic Examination
McRae R, 3rd edition, Churchill Livingstone, 1990.
A good guide to examining orthopaedic patients. Each step in the examination schemes is clearly illustrated with line drawings.

Concise System of Orthopaedics and Fractures
Apley AG and Solomon L, 2nd edition, Butterworth Heinemann, 1991.
A standard orthopaedics book, full of useful sketches, photographs and X-rays which bring the text to life. It contains examination schemes for different joints.

HOW TO USE THIS BOOK

This book consists of four sections. Sections I and II contain structured answer questions (SAQs) and answers. Sections III and IV contain essay questions and model answers.

Write your answers to the SAQs in the boxes provided. When you have finished, turn to Section II to mark your answers. Allow half marks for incomplete answers, and full marks for sensible and accurate alternatives that the authors have not considered. We hope that the examiners are equally understanding.

Every answer includes a short section of comments which provide concise teaching notes on each topic. Where necessary, refer to the list of recommended textbooks for further information.

At the back of the book, appendices B and C contain typical examination papers enabling you to gain experience of working under timed conditions. Twelve SAQs or four essay questions constitute a two-hour written paper.

Use the Revision Checklist provided to monitor your progress by ticking off subjects with which you feel confident.

SECTION I:
STRUCTURED ANSWER QUESTIONS

CHAPTER 1: SURGICAL PHYSIOLOGY

Question 1

A 49-year-old man with a history of macronodular cirrhosis is admitted for elective gastrointestinal surgery. His liver biochemistry is:

- **Conjugated bilirubin: 25 umol/l**
- **Alkaline phosphatase: 760 units/l**
- **Serum albumin: 15 g/l**
- **Aspartate and alanine amino transferases – elevated**
- **Plasma prothrombin index – decreased**
- **Gamma-glutamyl transferase – raised**

(a) Comment on his liver profile. (4 marks)

(b) How would you support his liver function prior to surgery? (3 marks)

Continues …

(c) List three surgical complications associated with the above dysfunction. (3 marks)

Question 2

A 67-year-old man with chronic lung disease is admitted for pre-operative assessment for elective abdominal surgery. His lung function tests are:

- **Peak expiratory flow rate (PEFR): 350 l/min (normal: 400–600 l/min)**
- **Forced expiratory volume in 1 second (FEV_1): 2.21 (normal: 3.21)**
- **Forced vital capacity (FVC): 4.21 (normal: 4.05.51)**
- **pO_2: 7.8 Kpa (normal: 10.6 Kpa)**
- **pCO_2: 6.98 Kpa (normal: 4.6–6.4 Kpa)**

(a) Comment on his respiratory impairment. (4 marks)

(b) Outline measures to improve lung function prior to surgery. (3 marks)

Continues …

(c) How would you support his respiratory function in the post-operative period? (3 marks)

Question 3

A 70-year-old man is assessed for an emergency laparotomy for peritonitis due to colonic diverticular perforation. He passes 45 ml of urine over the subsequent two hours; his peripheral blood count and serum biochemistry are:

- **Hb: 9.8 g/l**
- **WBC: 21.4 x 10^6 cells/cmm**
- **Na^+: 145 mmol/l**
- **K^+: 5.6 mmol/l**
- **HCO_3^-: 30 mmol/l**
- **Urea: 60 mmol/l**

(a) (i) Comment on his biochemical profile. (2 marks)
(ii) List the causes of the renal malfunction in this patient. (2 marks)

(b) Outline how renal function may be improved prior to surgery. (2 marks)

Continues ...

(c) State a renal complication of surgery and anaesthesia and outline your management. (4 marks)

Question 4

A 78-year-old man weighing 53 kg was admitted from a nursing home with a 14-day history of persistent vomiting. He was very dehydrated and malnourished.

(a) (i) How would you estimate his fluid and electrolyte deficit? (1 mark)
(ii) List the fluid and electrolyte preparations you would use, with their approximate compositions, to correct his deficit. (2 marks)
(iii) How would you monitor his fluid replacement therapy? (2 marks)

(b) (i) How would you assess his state of nutrition? (2 marks)
(ii) Discuss briefly how you would work out his protein and calorie requirements. (3 marks)

Question 5

A 65-year-old man is admitted with a three-day history of vomiting and a diagnosis of gastric outlet obstruction is made. He is placed on nasogastric aspiration and an IV infusion of 5% dextrose, alternating with Hartmann's (Ringer lactate) solution over the next 48 hours. His serum biochemistry on admission was Na^+ 120 mmol/L; K^+ 3.7 mmol/L, HCO_3^- 40 mmol/L. His urinary pH at the end of this period is 7.2.

(a) (i) State the biochemical diagnosis on admission. (1 mark)
(ii) Comment on the fluid and electrolyte replacement that followed. (3 marks)

(b) Write a note on the metabolic factors responsible for the production of acidic urine. (6 marks)

Question 6

A 60-year-old man underwent elective abdominal surgery for repair of an aortic aneurysm.

(a) (i) What is the metabolic response in respect to fluid and electrolyte balance in the first 24 hours of surgery? (2 marks)
(ii) How would you adjust the fluid and electrolyte requirements during this period? (2 marks)

(b) His urine output fell to below 30 ml/hr following surgery.
(i) How would you determine the cause of his oliguria? (4 marks)
(ii) What remedial measures would you take? (2 marks)

Question 7

An adult male became pyrexial and developed an erythematous skin rash during a blood transfusion following surgery.

(a) (i) What factors are involved in these reactions? (2 marks)
(ii) What measures would you take to counteract these complications? (2 marks)

(b) In the post-operative period the patient required a 10-unit blood transfusion.
(i) What is the effect of this transfusion on liver function and clotting factors? (2 marks)
(ii) What is the effect on plasma potassium and calcium levels and how would you achieve homeostasis of these ions in the plasma? (4 marks)

Question 8

A 34-year-old man with advanced infection with the human immunodeficiency virus (HIV) developed bowel obstruction which requires emergency surgery.

(a) (i) List the changes in the haematological or biochemical parameters that would, in the perioperative period, make him susceptible to haemorrhage. (2 marks)

(ii) List the haematological or biochemical changes in the perioperatiove period that would make him susceptible to infection. (3 marks)

(b) (i) State the measures taken to protect theatre personnel from accidental inoculation with the patient's body fluids with regard to wearing of protective garb. (2 marks)

(ii) What important measures should be taken with regard to safety in surgical instrument usage? (3 marks)

Question 9

A 43-year-old woman suffering from diabetes mellitus is admitted as an emergency with gangrene of the toes of her left foot. ABG estimation revealed a pH of 7.1 and a partial pressure of CO_2 of 6.8.

(a) (i) State the acid-base disorder present. (1 mark)
(ii) Give two causes for this. (2 marks)

(b) (i) State the further investigations you would request. (3 marks)
(ii) How would you manage the metabolic disorder? (4 marks)

Question 10

A 49-year-old man with a malignant stricture of the oesophagus had lost 20% of his normal body weight over a three-month period.

(a) (i) State the cause of his weight loss. (1 mark)
(ii) How would you categorise his nutritional state? (1 mark)
(iii) List two clinical findings that would reflect the nutritional state. (2 marks)

(b) (i) How would you improve his nutritional state? (3 marks)
(ii) How would you monitor your nutrition therapy? (3 marks)

CHAPTER 2: TRAUMA AND BURNS

Question 1

A 30-year-old man is brought to the Accident and Emergency department having sustained a closed head injury from a blow to the back of the head.

(a) How would you assess the level of consciousness? (2 marks)

(b) List the physical signs you would elicit to establish the extent of the intracranial injury. (3 marks)

(c) (i) List the types of intracranial bleeding that may be present and state one investigation that would demonstrate the lesion. (2 marks)
(ii) Write a short note on your management. (3 marks)

Question 2

A 23-year-old motorcyclist sustained chest injuries in a road accident and was air-lifted to the Accident and Emergency department.

(a) State your immediate measures to assess and maintain respiratory and circulatory function. (3 marks)

(b) Identify two immediately life-threatening intra-thoracic emergencies during your primary clinical survey. (2 marks)

(c) Write a note on the management of:
(i) An open chest wound. (2 marks)
(ii) An haemo-pneumothorax. (3 marks)

Question 3

A driver of a motor vehicle involved in a head-on collision with another vehicle was air-lifted to the Accident and Emergency department fully conscious and communicative but becoming increasingly breathless, with central cyanosis and bruising over his right upper chest.

(a) (i) State the two probable causes for his progressive respiratory failure. (2 marks)
(ii) List the clinical signs you would elicit to confirm your diagnoses. (2 marks)

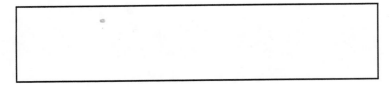

(b) (i) State one blood investigation you would urgently request. (1 mark)
(ii) State the radiological investigations that would confirm the diagnosis. (1 mark)

Continues …

(c) State four potentially lethal thoracic injuries he may have sustained which may not be apparent during the initial clinical survey. (4 marks)

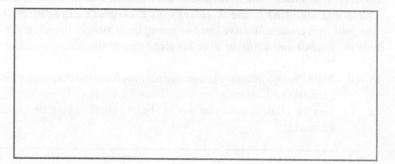

Question 4

A 43-year-old woman fell off her horse in a riding accident. She complains of severe and persistent upper abdominal pain radiating to her back.

(a) (i) List the possible intra-abdominal visceral injuries sustained. (2 marks)
(ii) State one non-invasive investigation you would perform to assess the presence and extent of an intra-abdominal injury. (1 mark)

(b) (i) How would you monitor this patient in the Accident and Emergency department? (2 marks)
(ii) What are the immediate resuscitatory measures you may be called upon to perform? (2 marks)

Continues …

(c) Discuss the clinical and other findings that would require an emergency surgical exploration of the abdomen. (3 marks)

Question 5

You are a member of an air ambulance team attending to a 28-year-old man with multiple injuries at the site of a road traffic accident.

(a) State in order of priority your measures to ensure patient survival until transfer to a trauma centre. (5 marks)

(b) The patient is trapped in the wreckage of his vehicle and his transfer is delayed by three hours. Discuss your supportive measures. (3 marks)

(c) List the ideal composition of an air ambulance team. (2 marks)

Question 6

An 18-year-old motor cyclist involved in a road traffic accident was admitted to the Accident and Emergency department. He is fully conscious but complained of severe neck pain.

(a) List the possible injuries to the cervical spine and cervical cord he may have sustained. (2 marks)

(b) When gently examining the neck:
   (i) What findings would suggest a spinal injury? (1 mark)
   (ii) What manoeuvre should you not perform? (1 mark)

(c) If he were found to have a spinal fracture and cord lesion at C5–T1 level:
   (i) Discuss your treatment of the injury. (2 marks)
   (ii) How would you prevent complications as a sequelae to the injury? (4 marks)

Question 7

An 8-year-old girl suffered hot water scalds to the whole of her chest and abdomen. She is admitted to the Accident and Emergency department conscious and very distressed.

(a) (i) How would you estimate the surface area affected? (1 mark)
(ii) State the immediate medical measures you would take. (4 marks)

(b) (i) How would you distinguish between a partial and a full thickness skin burn? (2 marks)
(ii) How would you calculate the fluid replacement for the first 24 hours? (3 marks)

Question 8

A 30-year-old secretary was rescued from an office fire. She is breathless and coughing, with traces of soot around her nose and mouth. She had suffered no external burns.

(a) (i) State the injury sustained. (1 mark)
(ii) Give your immediate resuscitation measures. (2 marks)

(b) She develops stridor and respiratory distress.
(i) State the pathological process involved. (2 marks)
(ii) How would you manage her airway? (2 marks)
(iii) How would you treat the injury sustained? (3 marks)

Question 9

A 20-year-old man injured his neck when the scrum collapsed on him while playing rugby.

(a) (i) How would you avoid compounding a suspected spinal injury? (2 marks)
(ii) How would you investigate for the integrity of the cervical spine? (2 marks)

(b) If the patient is unconscious list the clinical findings that suggest a cervical cord injury. (3 marks)

(c) Write a note on neurogenic shock following cervical cord injury. (3 marks)

Question 10

A 15-year-old cyclist was admitted to the Accident and Emergency department following a traffic accident. He is conscious but very pale, with bruising over the right lower chest and abdomen, and a swelling of the right thigh and knee.

(a) How would you assess for the following:
   (i) Lung injury. (2 marks)
   (ii) Intra-abdominal injury. (2 marks)
   (iii) Lower limb injury. (2 marks)

(b) He develops hypovolaemic shock. List your immediate measures to resuscitate him. (4 marks)

Question 11

A 5-year-old boy was seen in the Accident and Emergency department, having sustained hot water scalds to his arms, chest and abdomen at home.

(a) How would you determine on examination the extent and depth of his wounds? (3 marks)

(b) State your criteria for admission. (3 marks)

(c) Write a note on the methods of dressing his wounds. (4 marks)

Question 12

A 38-year-old railway worker is admitted to the Accident and Emergency department with electrical burns to his back and arm, from contact with high tension overhead conductors.

(a) State three urgent priorities in his clinical assessment. (3 marks)

(b) Write a note on the type of burn injury sustained. (3 marks)

(c) Discuss the effect of the injury on the heart, kidneys, skeletal muscle and nervous system. (4 marks)

Question 13

A 49-year-old motorist sustained burns to 35% of his body surface from burning fuel in a traffic accident.

(a) How would you estimate his fluid requirements for the first 24 hours? (3 marks)

(b) What measures would you take to prevent wound infection? (4 marks)

(c) How would you manage a non-survivable burn injury? (3 marks)

Question 14

Five patients injured in a single motor vehicle accident are admitted to the Accident and Emergency Department. They are:

- **Patient 1: an 18-year-old front-seat passenger found 10 m from the vehicle. He is awake and complains of severe chest and limb pains; there are angulated deformities of the left forearm and left thigh; his BP is 90/60, pulse 140 bpm and respiration 35/min**
- **Patient 2: a 19-year-old male, found in the driving seat of the vehicle, is unconscious with severe facial bruising and bleeding from the nose and mouth; there are multiple abrasions over the anterior chest wall; his BP is 150/80, pulse 120 bpm and respiration 40/min**
- **Patient 3: a 20-year-old hysterical woman extracted from the floor of the back seat complains of abdominal pains; she is eight months pregnant and is found to be active labout; her vital signs are normal**
- **Patient 4: a 16-year-old girl, a back-seat passenger, complains of severe neck pain and paraesthesia of both arms and hands; her vital signs are normal**
- **Patient 5: a 17-year-old girl, a back-seat passenger, complains of pain in her right hip and both feet; she has bruising and deformities of both ankles; her vital signs are normal**

(a) In what order would you care for these patients? Place them in descending order of priority. (3 marks)

Continues ...

(b) Briefly outline your reasons for prioritizing the patients thus. (7 marks)

Question 15

A hurricane with heavy rains caused a mud slide, burying a section of a hillside village. Five villagers were rescued 18 hours later. They are:

- **Patient 1: a 44-year-old man found buried in mud; he is comatose with weak peripheral pulses, there are open wounds over the shoulder and back which are not actively bleeding**
- **Patient 2: a 34-year-old woman who fell 10 m down a precipice; she is awake but very lethargic with a large laceration in her scalp that is actively bleeding**
- **Patient 3: a 13-year-old girl found pinned under a fallen tree; she is awake and alert and complains of pain in both legs and numbness of her feet; she has swelling, bruising and angulated deformities of the right knee and left leg**
- **Patient 4: a 29-year-old woman who dug herself out from under the mud, is increasingly breathless and complains of right-sided chest and abdominal pain; paradoxical movement is observed over the right chest**
- **Patient 5: a nine-year-old girl found wandering near the mud slide, is distressed and confused but appears not to be in pain and to have no external injuries**

(a) In what order would you care for these patients? Place them in descending order of priority. (3 marks)

(b) Briefly outline your reasons for prioritizing the patients thus. (7 marks)

Question 16

Five holidaymakers were admitted to the Accident and Emergency Department two hours following a gas cylinder explosion and fire in a caravan at a seaside resort. They are:

- **Patient 1: a 38-year-old man with 60% full and partial thickness surface burns to the anterior aspect of his torso and limbs; he has a large laceration in the scalp and is expectorating carbonaceous sputum; his BP is 130/100, pulse 120/min and respiration 30/min**
- **Patient 2: a 32-year-old woman with 25% ful and partial thickness burns to the chest and arms and forearms complains of severe neck pains and has bruising and a deformity of her left shoulder; her BP is 120/90, pulse 100/min and respiration 28/min**
- **Patient 3: a 72-year-old woman with 65% surface burns to the face, chest, upper abdomen and arms is semi-comatose with sonorous breathing; her BP is 110/90, pulse 125/min and respiration 14/min**
- **Patient 4: a 12-year-old boy with 15% mostly superficial burns is found to have deep lacerations to his left hip and thigh which are actively bleeding; his BP is 90/60, pulse 130/min and respiration 28/min**
- **Patient 5: a five-year-old girl was found confused and lethargic with soot over her nose and mouth and had sustained no external injuries; her BP is 110/70, pulse 110/min and respiration 32/min**

(a) In what order would you care for these patients? Place them in descending order of priority. (3 marks)

(b) Briefly outline your reasons for prioritizing the patients thus. (7 marks)

Question 17

You are the casualty officer in an Accident and Emergency Department when you are informed by the police that a passenger aircraft has overshot the runway on landing and caught fire at the local airport 15 miles away. Casualties are being taken to three hospitals in the area and you are to expect the arrival of some of them.

(a) List the hospital personnel you need to contact immediately. (3 marks)

(b) List the parts of the hospital you would designate as reception and treatment areas. (3 marks)

(c) What categories of triage would you use for the incoming casualties? (4 marks)

CHAPTER 3: ORTHOPAEDICS

Question 1

A 14-year-old child presents with pain over a swelling of three months' duration, arising from the lower end of the femur.

(a) State two investigations that would assist in the diagnosis.

(b) List three bone tumours that may present at this age. (3 marks)

(c) Outline the principles of treating bone tumours in childhood. (5 marks)

Question 2

A 33-year-old otherwise health woman presents with a nine-month history of progressive pain in her lower back which is worse following activity; over the past few weeks she developed tingling sensations and numbness in the left leg.

(a) Outline the probable cause of her symptoms and state the likely diagnosis. (3 marks)

(b) How would you identify the site of the lesion by neurological assessement? (3 marks)

(c) Outline the principles of treating this condition. (4 marks)

Question 3

A 69-year-old woman develops increasing pain and stiffness in the hip six months after hip joint replacement on that side.

(a) List three causes for her symptoms. (3 marks)

(b) How would you assess her symptoms? (3 marks)

(c) Outline the factors that contribute to the complications of joint replacement surgery. (4 marks)

Question 4

A 61-year-old woman complains of swelling, pain and inflammation of her bunions which for many years have been the cause of unsightly deformity of her feet.

(a) (i) State your diagnosis. (2 marks)
(ii) List the factors responsible for her symptoms. (2 marks)

(b) State the predisposing cause of this deformity. (2 marks)

(c) Outline the surgical treatment of this condition. (4 marks)

Question 5

A 44-year-old woman gives a six-month history of progressive pain in her neck on movement, following a mild whip-lash injury. In recent weeks she has experienced numbness and weakness in her right hand.

(a) State the probable diagnosis and the causative factors. (3 marks)

(b) How would you assess the segmental level of the neurological lesion? (3 marks)

(c) Outline the principles of treating this condition. (4 marks)

Question 6

A 9-year-old schoolgirl presents at the orthopaedic clinic with a 4-month history of pain in her left groin and hip, and a progressive limp. She gives history of trauma or other symptoms.

(a) List the positive findings you would expect on examining her hip. (3 marks)

(b) (i) State two diseases that may present thus at this age. (2 marks)
(ii) List the radiological features you would expect to see in each. (2 marks)

(c) What are their complications if left untreated? (3 marks)

Question 7

A 17-year-old schoolboy sustained an external rotational injury to his right ankle during a rugby tackle. There was considerable pain, bruising and swelling.

(a) List the possible injuries to the ankle. (4 marks)

(b) Radiology of the ankle and distal tibia and fibula showed no fracture. What related bony and/or ligamentous injuries would you wish to exclude? (2 marks)

(c) Write a note on the treatment of an unstable ankle injury. (4 marks)

Question 8

A 40-year-old woman suffered with pain, swelling and loss of mobility in her fingers, which over a period of time affected her wrists and feet.

(a) (i) State the likely diagnosis. (1 mark)

(ii) Write a note on the pathological changes in the joints. (3 marks)

(b) List the positive blood investigations in this disease. (3 marks)

(c) State the principles of management. (3 marks)

Question 9

A 64-year-old woman with pain, stiffness and limitation of movement in her left hip is diagnosed as having osteoarthritis.

(a) List the radiological features in the hip joint. (3 marks)

(b) State non-surgical measures to alleviate symptoms and preserve function. (3 marks)

(c) (i) List the indications for operative treatment. (3 marks)
(ii) State the operation of choice for this patient. (1 mark)

Question 10

A 6-year-old boy sustained a supracondylar fracture to his right arm during a fall in the school playground.

(a) Write a note on the treatment of the fracture. (4 marks)

(b) Eight hours after the fracture was reduced the child is crying with severe pain and was unable to grasp objects with the right hand. The forearm is swollen and the radial pulse absent. Write a note on your diagnosis and treatment. (3 marks)

(c) List the complications of this fracture. (3 marks)

Question 11

(a) Write a note on how you would diagnose and treat congenital dislocation of the hip in the neonatal period. (5 marks)

(b) List the factors which give rise to this condition. (2 marks)

(c) If the diagnosis is delayed until the child starts walking, discuss the treatment options and prognosis. (3 marks)

Question 12

A child of 5 years presents to her family practitioner with a 3-day history of severe pain in her left forearm, with fever and malaise. The forearm is inflamed and swollen.

(a) (i) State the probable diagnosis. (1 mark)

(ii) Write a note on the investigations that would aid the diagnosis. (3 marks)

(b) Give three differential diagnoses of the forearm swelling. (3 marks)

(c) Outline your treatment. (3 marks)

Question 13

A boy of 8 years is referred from a child welfare clinic with a growth curve well below the normal range. Clinically there is thickening of his wrists and ankles, and bowing of his legs.

(a) (i) State the likely clinical diagnosis. (1 mark)
(ii) List the radiological features which would confirm your diagnosis. (2 marks)
(iii) List the biochemical features which would confirm your diagnosis. (2 marks)

(b) (i) State the causative factors. (3 marks)
(ii) Outline the treatment. (2 marks)

Question 14

A 60-year-old man presents with long-standing dull pain in his back and hips, and is found to be of short stature, with kyphosis of the spine and slight forward bowing of his legs.

(a) (i) State the probable clinical diagnosis. (1 mark)
(ii) Discuss the bony changes that characterize this disease. (4 marks)

(b) List four complications of this disease. (2 marks)

(c) Write a note on the principles of treatment. (3 marks)

Question 15

A 47-year-old factory worker presents with a painless, fluctuant swelling in his right groin. A kyphotic angulation of the dorsal spine is observed on examination.

(a) (i) State the probable diagnosis. (1 mark)
(ii) Discuss the pathological basis of the clinical findings. (2 marks)

(b) List the investigations to confirm your diagnosis. (3 marks)

Continues …

(c) (i) Discuss your objectives in treatment. (3 marks)
(ii) State a serious complication that may be precipitated in this patient. (1 mark)

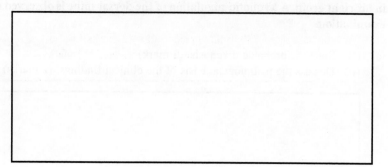

Question 16

A 5-year-old child suffering from protein-calorie malnutrition presents with an inflamed, swollen and painful forearm of four days' duration.

(a) (i) State two lesions that may present thus. (2 marks)
(ii) How would movements in that limb be affected? (2 marks)

(b) (i) List the common organisms that are implicated. (2 marks)
(ii) Discuss the treatment of these two lesions. (4 marks)

CHAPTER 4: NEUROSURGERY

Question 1

A 31-year-old man, a known HIV carrier, gives a six-month history of recurrent episodes of paranasal sinusitus and, more recently, of febrile episodes and severe headaches. Clinically, he is found to have right oculomotor nerve palsy, loss of positional sense and an unstable gait.

(a) State the probable diagnosis and the cause of his most recent symptoms. (3 marks)

(b) State one investigation that would confirm your diagnosis and localize the lesion. (2 marks)

Continues ...

(c) Outline the treatment of this condition. (5 marks)

Question 2

A 40-year-old merchant seaman with a five-month history of headaches, paraesthesia and progressive weakness in his left lower limb is found to have a glial tumour of the right cerebral hemisphere.

(a) List four glial tumours. (2 marks)

(b) State a method of confirming the diagnosis. (2 marks)

(c) Outline the principles of treating cerebral tumours. (6 marks)

Question 3

A 37-year-old bookmaker gives a seven-year history of fits, associated with blackouts, followed by transient loss of speech and cognitive function, which are poorly controlled on anti-epileptic medical treatment.

(a) List three investigations that may localize the seizure focus. (3 marks)

(b) State the indications for surgical treatment. (4 marks)

(c) How would you counsel the patient for seizure sugery? (3 marks)

Question 4

An 11-month-old male infant was referred to the Neurosurgical Clinic with a history of failure to thrive and achieve milestones. A progressive increase in skull circumference had been noted since birth.

(a) (i) State the likely diagnosis. (1 mark)
(ii) What are the positive clinical findings? (2 marks)
(iii) State one important investigation to confirm your diagnosis. (1 mark)

(b) (i) State a common cause for this condition. (1 mark)
(ii) Give two associated malformations of the central nervous system. (2 marks)

(c) Write a note on the definitive treatment for this condition. (3 marks)

Question 5

A 48-year-old woman with a nine-month history of epileptic fits and headaches is found to have focal neurological signs and papilloedema.

(a) (i) State your working diagnosis. (1 mark)
(ii) Discuss briefly the pathophysiology of the abnormal findings. (3 marks)

(b) (i) State two investigations that would reveal the lesion. (2 marks)
(ii) Why would a lumbar puncture be contraindicated? (1 mark)

(c) List three benign and three malignant lesions that would present thus. (3 marks)

Question 6

A previously healthy 32-year-old woman was admitted complaining of sudden onset of severe headache, with nausea and vomiting. She was found to be drowsy with neck stiffness.

(a) (i) State the likely diagnosis and the underlying lesion. (2 marks)
(ii) If her condition deteriorates, state the progressive changes in the clinical findings. (3 marks)

(b) (i) State one non-invasive investigation to confirm your diagnosis. (1 mark)
(ii) State your findings on lumbar puncture. (1 mark)

Continues …

(c) Write a note on her management. (3 marks)

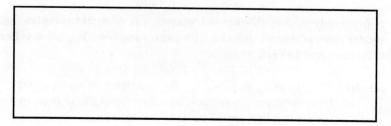

Question 7

A conscious 75-year-old woman is admitted with a left hemisphere stroke.

(a) (i) List three prime neurological findings. (2 marks)
(ii) List four risk factors of stroke. (2 marks)

(b) The patient's condition deteriorates; outline your immediate management. (6 marks)

Question 8

A 6-year-old child presents with fever and fits. A cranial CT scan revealed a brain abscess.

(a) How would you arrive at this diagnosis clinically? (3 marks)

(b) (i) List four causative organisms. (2 marks)
(ii) List two underlying sources of infection that predispose to brain abscess in this child. (2 marks)

(c) Write a note on specific treatment. (3 marks)

Question 9

A 56-year-old woman complains of gradual onset of pain in her neck, radiating down her left arm. She also experienced tingling down the limb during neck extension.

(a) List three lesions of the spinal cord and three lesions of the cervical spine that may give rise to her symptoms. (3 marks)

(b) Write a note on the likely neurological findings. (3 marks)

(c) (i) List the radiological investigations to confirm your diagnosis. (2 marks)
(ii) State the principles of treatment. (2 marks)

CHAPTER 5: EYES, ENT AND SKIN

Question 1

An 8-year-old eastern European child is air-lifted from a refugee camp for the treatment of an ulcerating lesion in her left cheek exposing the buccal cavity and the alveolar margin.

(a) State your diagnosis. (2 marks)

(b) List the aetiological factors implicated in its causation. (3 marks)

(c) Outline your treatment priorities in the management of this condition. (5 marks)

Question 2

An 11-year-old boy with a four-year history of recurrent throat infections presents to the Accident and Emergency Department with fever, malaise, sore throat and dysphagia.

(a) (i) State the probable diagnosis. (2 marks)
(ii) What is a frequently accompanying lesion in the nasopharynx? (2 marks)

(b) List the findings on examination. (3 marks)

(c) Outline the definitive treatment for these lesions. (3 marks)

Question 3

A 7-year-old child in equatorial Africa is seen by you during your overseas elective spell with a four-month history of a minimally symptomatic swelling over the cheek bone, deforming her face.

(a) (i) State your probable diagnosis. (2 marks)
(ii) Give two investigations to confirm your diagnosis. (2 marks)

(b) List the aetiological factors associated with this condition. (3 marks)

(c) How would you treat this lesion? (3 marks)

Question 4

A 38-year-old man presents with an unhealed ulcer over a burn scar over the left shin that he sustained two years previously

(a) State the likely diagnosis and your clinical findings. (4 marks)

(b) How would you confirm your diagnosis? (2 marks)

(c) How would you treat this lesion? (4 marks)

Question 5

A 70-year-old woman suffered a sudden painless loss of vision in one eye.

(a) Give four possible causes. (4 marks)

(b) State three associated systemic diseases. (3 marks)

(c) If she had suffered loss of vision in both eyes, state two probable causes. (3 marks)

Question 6

A 3-year-old toddler is seen in the Accident and Emergency department with a 5-day history of a painful red eye.

(a) List four possible causes. (2 marks)

(b) Write a note on your examination of the eye. (4 marks)

(c) If a white pupillary reflex was seen on fundoscopy, state your probable diagnosis and management. (4 marks)

Question 7

An 11-year-old boy was admitted with right-sided proptosis, oedematous conjunctivitis (chemosis) and reduced visual acuity. He was found to be pyrexial, dehydrated and lethargic. There was a recent history of recurrent acute sinus infection.

(a) (i) State your clinical diagnosis. (1 mark)
(ii) What microbiological and radiological investigations would you request? (2 marks)

(b) (i) State your medical management of this condition. (2 marks)
(ii) How would you monitor the response to your medical measures? (2 marks)

Continues …

(c) The child fails to improve, with deterioration in his eye signs. A CT scan shows an opacity of the right maxillary sinus and an abscess under the orbital plate of the ethmoid bone.

(i) State the surgical measures required. (2 marks)
(ii) State a potentially lethal complication of this condition. (1 mark)

Question 8

A cricketer fielding close to the wicket was struck in the orbit by a firmly hit cricket ball. He presented to the Accident and Emergency department with periocular ecchymosis and periorbital swelling.

(a) (i) State the probable orbital injury sustained. (1 mark)
(ii) State the mechanism of the injury to the orbit. (2 marks)

(b) (i) Discuss the positive findings when examining for orbital damage. (3 marks)
(ii) List the investigations you would require to exclude bony injury. (1 mark)

(c) Discuss the principles of managing this injury. (3 marks)

Question 9

A 48-year-old man presents to the ENT clinic with a six-week history of progressive hoarseness not responding to antibiotics.

(a) List four non-malignant lesions of the vocal cords that may present thus. (2 marks)

(b) Write a note on two methods of clinically examining the larynx. (4 marks)

(c) A biopsy of a small lesion on the vocal cord revealed a squamous cell carcinoma (glottic carcinoma). Discuss the treatment options available. (4 marks)

Question 10

A 5-year-old boy was referred from the school clinic with a persistent hearing loss in one ear. A diagnosis of 'glue ear' was made.

(a) (i) Discuss the nature of the hearing loss. (2 marks)
(ii) List three predisposing factors. (2 marks)

(b) Describe the appearance of the ear drum in this condition. (2 marks)

(c) Discuss two methods of surgically treating this condition. (4 marks)

Question 11

A 54-year old woman presents with a 12-week history of a circumscribed 2.5cm diameter itchy, ulcerating pigmented skin lesion on her upper back; it had recently bled.

(a) (i) What are the other clinical features of the lesion you would look for on examination? (1 mark)
(ii) State a malignant lesion that may present thus. (1 mark)
(iii) How is it staged histologically? (2 marks)

(b) How would you treat this lesion? (3 marks)

(c) Write a short note on the public health measures you would adopt to reduce the incidence of this form of skin cancer in the community. (3 marks)

Question 12

A small, circumscribed raised lesion on the cheek of an 87-year-old woman bled following minor trauma.

(a) State three malignant lesions that may present thus. (3 marks)

(b) If your clinical diagnosis is a form of skin cancer, what are the treatment options available? (4 marks)

(c) (i) Discuss the association of solar radiation with the development of skin lesions. (2 marks)
(ii) What protective measures would you advise? (1 mark)

CHAPTER 6: ENDOCRINOLOGY, BREAST AND CHEST

Question 1

A 35-year-old woman presents to the surgical clinic with a gradually enlarging asymptomatic swelling in the front of her neck.

(a) (i) State the structures likely to be involved. (2 marks)
(ii) How would you clinically distinguish one from the other? (2 marks)

(b) Discuss the investigations you would perform to confirm your clinical impression. (2 marks)

(c) If you had diagnosed a goitre, state the clinical findings that would require surgical intervention. (4 marks)

Question 2

A 30-year-old woman presents to the surgical clinic with symptoms of restlessness, insomnia and a preference to cooler weather. She has a pulse rate of 110 per minute and a painless swelling of her thyroid gland.

(a) (i) State your probable diagnosis. (1 mark)
(ii) List other clinical features that would support this diagnosis. (3 marks)

(b) State the investigations you would perform to assess her thyroid function. (3 marks)

(c) Discuss the management of this condition. (3 marks)

Question 3

A 64-year-old woman presents to the surgical clinic with a long-standing thyroid swelling, complaining of recent onset of pain in the neck and hoarseness.

(a) Write a short note on the clinical findings that would assist you in reaching a diagnosis. (3 marks)

(b) State the probable cause of the hoarseness and the examination you would carry out to confirm this. (2 marks)

(c) (i) State the investigations you would request to confirm your clinical diagnosis. (3 marks)
(ii) What is referred to as a 'cold nodule' on thyroid imaging? (2 marks)

Question 4

A 46-year-old woman in chronic renal failure sustained a pathological fracture of her hip.

(a) Discuss briefly the metabolic basis for the fracture. (3 marks)

(b) Her serum parathyroid hormone (PTH) titres were raised. Explain the parathyroid hyperfunction in relation to renal failure. (3 marks)

(c) State how you would counteract the elevated PTH titres. (4 marks)

Question 5

A 25-year-old, otherwise healthy woman gives a 12-month history of headaches of increasing frequency, accompanied by flushes and sweats. Her BP is 180/120 and a CT scan of her abdomen reveals a right-sided adrenal tumour measuring 5.5 cm in size. Her 24-hour urinary metanephrines and vanillyl mandelic acid levels were significantly raised.

(a) (i) State the likely diagnosis. (1 mark)
    (ii) What other biochemical test(s) would confirm your diagnosis? (2 marks)

(b) (i) Discuss the functional disorders caused by this lesion (2 marks)
    (ii) Give the medical management of these. (3 marks)
    (iii) State the definitive treatment for this disease. (2 marks)

Question 6

A 58-year-old woman presents with a nine-month history of progressive fatigue, weight gain and spontaneous skin bruising. She was found to be hypertensive, with impaired glucose tolerance.

(a) (i) State the endocrine disorder. (1 mark)
(ii) Name one laboratory investigation that would confirm your diagnosis. (1 mark)

(b) (i) State the source of this disease. (1 mark)
(ii) Give one investigation to define the anatomical site of the lesion. (1 mark)
(iii) List three other endocrine disorders that may arise from the same gland. (3 marks)

(c) Discuss the principles of treating this patient. (3 marks)

Question 7

A worried 46-year-old woman, attending the Breast Clinic, gives a three-week history of a blood-stained discharge from her right nipple.

(a) (i) List three possible abnormal findings during your examination of her breast. (2 marks)

(ii) List other anatomical regions you would include in your examination. (2 marks)

(iii) List three clinical diagnoses you would consider. (3 marks)

(b) List three specific investigations that would assist you in arriving at a diagnosis. (3 marks)

Question 8

An anxious 36-year-old woman, attending the Breast Clinic, gives a two-week history of an asymptomatic lump in her left breast.

(a) (i) List the clinical characteristics of the presenting lesion. (2 marks)
(ii) State the sites of lymphatic drainage of the breast. (2 marks)

(b) List the investigations that would assist in confirming your clinical diagnosis. (2 marks)

(c) List the treatment modalities available for breast malignancy. (4 marks)

Question 9

A 78-year-old woman presents to the Breast Clinic with an asymptomatic, hard and irregular mobile lump in her right breast.

(a) (i) State the most likely histological diagnosis. (1 mark)
(ii) How would you assess distant spread? (3 marks)

(b) The lump has been present for over six years with little alteration in size
(i) Is the diagnosis of malignancy still likely? (1 mark)
(ii) How would you treat her if malignancy is confirmed? (2 marks)
(iii) If she declines your offer of treatment, what would be the likely outcome? (3 marks)

Question 10

A 55-year-old woman is referred to the Breast Clinic following a screening mammography.

(a) State three investigations you would perform on a barely palpable right-sided breast lump. (3 marks)

(b) The lump is removed under stereotactic guidance and was found to be a lobular carcinoma with vascular invasion. List your investigations for the presence of distant metastases. (3 marks)

(c) State the principles of treatment. (4 marks)

Question 11

An 18-month-old boy presents with episodes of breathlessness and cyanosis, usually following feeds; there is no history of vomiting. On examination bowel sounds are heard over his left chest wall.

(a) (i) State your working diagnosis. (1 mark)
    (ii) List the radiological findings on CXR. (3 marks)

(b) List the complications of delayed diagnosis. (3 marks)

(c) State the principles of surgical treatment. (3 marks)

Question 12

A 46-year-old man gives a four-month history of cough and breathlessness, with right-sided chest pain. A thoracoscopy is arranged.

(a) Write a short note on this procedure. (3 marks)

(b) An empyema thoracis is diagnosed; state how you would manage this condition. (4 marks)

(c) List the aetiological factors associated with this diagnosis. (3 marks)

Question 13

A 71-year-old woman who is a long-term smoker presents with an enlarged asymptomatic lymph node at the root of her neck.

(a) List four malignant diseases that may present thus. (2 marks)

(b) Biopsy of the node reveals a deposit of small cell carcinoma. State your clinical diagnosis and the investigations to confirm this. (4 marks)

(c) State the principles of surgical treatment of this lesion. (4 marks)

Question 14

A 69-year old pensioner suffers from angina of effort which had progressively worsened over a 20-month period despite medical measures to control his symptoms.

(a) (i) State your probable diagnosis. (1 mark)
 (ii) State two non-invasive investigations to confirm your diagnosis. (1 mark)
 (iii) What information would be obtained therefrom? (2 marks)

(b) (i) Write a note on the radiological method used to investigate and treat this disease. (3 marks)

(c) Write a note on the principles of surgical treatment of this disease. (3 marks)

CHAPTER 7: UPPER ALIMENTARY TRACT

Question 1

A 43-year-old man gives a four-month history of dyspepsia, abdominal distention and weight loss. He is of pallid complexion with negative abdominal findings; however, a lymph node was palpable in the left supraventricular fossa.

(a) State the significance of the enlarged node and how it would assist in arriving at a diagnosis. (2 marks)

(b) List three investigations you would perform. (3 marks)

(c) State three types of gastric cancer and outline the principles of treatment. (5 marks)

Question 2

A 40-year-old man presents to the surgical clinic with a two-year history of an asymptomatic, slow-growing firm lump on the side of his face just below the lobe of his ear.

(a) (i) State the likely diagnosis. (1 mark)
    (ii) List the characteristics of the lesion you would ascertain on examination. (3 marks)

(b) A request was made for cytological confirmation by percutaneous needle biopsy of the lesion. Give your comments. (2 marks)

(c) (i) Write a note on the principles of surgical treatment. (3 marks)
(ii) What structures must be preserved from injury? (1 mark)

Question 3

A 29-year-old man is referred to the Accident and Emergency Department with a 10-day history of progressive pain and swelling of the floor of his mouth and upper part of his neck. He was pyrexial, with inflamed palpable nodes in the neck.

(a) (i) State the likely diagnosis and the anatomic planes involved in the inflammatory process. (2 marks)
(ii) List the pathogenic organisms that are associated with this lesion. (2 marks)

(b) (i) What are the consequences if left untreated? (2 marks)
(ii) How would you treat this lesion? (4 marks)

Question 4

A 71-year old man is referred to the surgical clinic with increasing difficulty in swallowing and significant weight loss over a period of six months.

(a) What other aspects of the history would assist you in arriving at a clinical diagnosis? (2 marks)

(b) (i) List the possible causes of dysphagia in this patient. (3 marks)
(ii) Name two investigations which would confirm your clinical diagnosis; what information would you obtain from each? (2 marks)

(c) Write a note on the aetiological factors associated with any two diagnoses. (3 marks)

Question 5

A 40-year-old male business executive presents with a six-month history of upper abdominal pain that comes on in the evenings and wakes him up in the early hours of the morning. Symptoms are relieved by food, milk and antacids.

(a) (i) State your clinical diagnosis. (1 mark)
(ii) Discuss briefly the aetiological factors that are associated with this disease. (2 marks)

(b) State one investigation that would demonstrate both the site and appearance of the lesion, and write a note on how this investigation is performed. (2 marks)

(c) (i) Discuss briefly the principles of treating this disease. (3 marks)
(ii) List the complications of this disease. (2 marks)

Question 6

A 4-month-old infant is referred with a history of projectile vomiting and poor weight gain since birth. His mother had felt a lump in his abdomen following feeds.

(a) (i) State your working diagnosis. (2 marks)
(ii) List two differential diagnoses. (2 marks)
(iii) What is the nature of the lump that the mother felt? (1 mark)

(b) Write a short note on the pathophysiology of this lesion. (2 marks)

(c) Discuss the principles of treatment. (3 marks)

Question 7

A newborn baby was found to regurgitate his feeds and developed a post-aspiration respiratory infection.

(a) (i) State your working diagnosis. (1 mark)
(ii) State the radiological investigation required to confirm your diagnosis. (1 mark)

(b) (i) Write a note or illustrate the congenital malformations that may present thus. (4 marks)
(ii) State a simple procedure that could be performed at birth to exclude this abnormality. (2 marks)

(c) What are the principles of treatment? (2 marks)

Question 8

A 34-year-old otherwise healthy woman gives a history of heartburn and belching with waterbrash.

(a) (i) State your probable diagnosis. (1 mark)
(ii) Write a short note on the underlying lesion. (3 marks)
(iii) State one investigation you would perform to confirm your diagnosis. (1 mark)

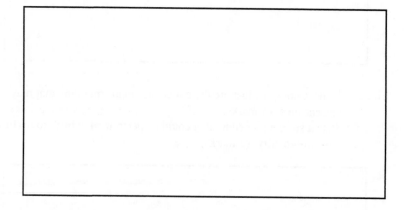

(b) (i) Discuss briefly the measures you would advise to alleviate her symptoms. (2 marks)
(ii) State the surgical procedures that would effect a cure. (3 marks)

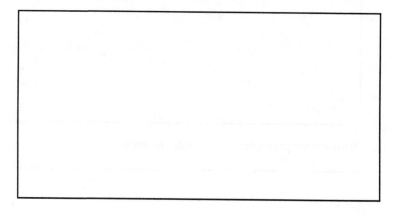

Question 9

A 39-year-old man with a six-month history of dyspepsia unresponsive to antacids is found to have an apparently normal gastric mucosa on endoscopy.

(a) List the tests you would perform on antral mucosal biopsies obtained in order to reach a diagnosis. (3 marks)

(b) (i) If a bacterial presence was detected, state the probable diagnosis. (1 mark)

(ii) How would you treat this infection? (3 marks)

(c) Write a note on the association of this pathogen with lesions of the stomach and duodenum. (3 marks)

Question 10

A 38-year-old man presents to the Accident and Emergency Department vomiting blood. An emergency upper GI endoscopy revealed bleeding from oesophageal varices.

(a) How would you control the bleeding? (4 marks)

(b) State the pathophysiology of this condition. (3 marks)

(c) What would be your follow-up protocol for this patient? (3 marks)

Question 11

A 36-year-old woman on anti-inflammatory medication for symptoms of rheumatoid arthritis developed severe upper abdominal pain of sudden onset. She is found to be pyrexial with a rigid abdomen.

(a) (i) State the probable diagnosis. (2 marks)
(ii) List the radiological features to confirm your diagnosis. (2 marks)

(b) Write a note on your treatment measures, including surgical measures if appropriate. (4 marks)

(c) State your measures to prevent recurrence of this disease. (2 marks)

Question 12

A 32-year-old man underwent an elective splenectomy for hypersplenism.

(a) List the three main types of post-operative bleeding in this patient. (3 marks)

(b) How would you manage such a haemorrhage in the immediate post-operative period? (4 marks)

(c) State the factors that may increase his susceptibility to infections, and your preventive measures. (3 marks)

Question 13

A 76-year-old man complains of a sore tongue. On examination a 1 cm ulcer was present on the postero-lateral aspect on the tongue with a patchy, white hyperkeratotic discoloration of the surrounding mucosa.

(a) List the clinical findings that would suggest a malignant ulcer. (3 marks)

(b) What is the surrounding mucosal lesion called? List the aetiological factors associated with this lesion. (3 marks)

(c) The ulcer on the tongue was found to be a squamous carcinoma. Discuss the principles of treatment. (4 marks)

CHAPTER 8: LIVER, GALL BLADDER AND PANCREAS

Question 1

A 16-year-old boy, a recent visitor to this country, is found to be moderately pale, febrile and having a large and tender spleen.

(a) List six causes of a chronically enlarged spleen. (3 marks)

(b) What do you understand by the term 'hypersplenism'? (3 marks)

(c) Outline the indications for splenectomy in this patient. (4 marks)

Question 2

A 40-year-old housewife complains of severe right upper abdominal pain radiating to the back, two hours after eating fried food.

(a) (i) Give your working diagnosis. (1 mark)
(ii) Give three physical signs you would expect to support this diagnosis. (2 marks)
(iii) Give one non-invasive investigation to support your diagnosis. (1 mark)

(b) Write a note on the pathogenesis of the disease. (3 marks)

(c) Discuss briefly the principles of surgical treatment. (3 marks)

Question 3

A 66-year-old woman with a history of calculus cholecystitis is admitted as an emergency feeling acutely ill, with progressive jaundice, right upper quadrant pain and rigors over the previous 3 days.

(a) (i) State your probable diagnosis. (1 mark)
(ii) Outline the causation and pathogenesis of this condition. (2 marks)
(iii) State the immediate blood investigations you would request, giving the reason for each. (3 marks)

(b) State two non-invasive methods of visualising the biliary tree in order to confirm your diagnosis. (1 mark)

(c) Discuss the principles of treatment. (3 marks)

Question 4

A 34-year-old woman became progressively jaundiced soon after an elective cholecystectomy.

(a) (i) State the most likely cause of her jaundice. (1 mark)
(ii) State an invasive investigation that would confirm your diagnosis. (1 mark).
(iii) How would you prepare the patient for this procedure? (2 marks)

(b) She develops a tender abdomen with rebound, rigors and a raised white blood cell count. State your diagnosis. (2 marks)

(c) Write a note on the measures the surgeon should adopt to avoid these complications. (4 marks)

Question 5

A 38-year-old woman presents acutely with symptoms of small bowel obstruction. She gave a six-month history of fatty food intolerance and upper right-sided abdominal pain with mild episodes of jaundice.

(a) (i) State the likely diagnosis. (1 mark)
(ii) What is the pathogenesis of the disease? (1 mark)
(iii) List the salient features on the AXR. (2 marks)

(b) How would you treat her bowel obstruction? (3 marks)

(c) Write a short note on your management of the underlying pathology. (3 marks)

Question 6

A 48-year-old woman presents with severe upper abdominal pain and vomiting. On examination, her abdomen is rigid and tender. A erect AXR was normal. Both serum amylase titres and white cell count were raised.

(a) (i) State the probable diagnosis. (1 mark)
(ii) Give two main causes for this condition. (2 marks)

(b) Outline your management. (4 marks)

(c) List the complications of this disease. (3 marks)

Question 7

A 78-year-old man gives a six-week history of progressive jaundice, anorexia and weight loss. Clinically he is malnourished and pale, and abdominal examination revealed a palpable gall bladder and a liver edge.

(a) State the probable diagnosis and list the investigations you would require to confirm it. (3 marks)

(b) (i) List your treatment options for this patient. (3 marks)
(ii) What factors would decide against major curative surgery? (2 marks)

(c) If the patient underwent an abdominal operation, list the post-operative complications that are associated with jaundice. (2 marks)

Question 8

A 15-year-old boy sustained blunt injury to the liver and pancreas in a traffic accident; he underwent surgical repair of a laceration to the right lobe of the liver and drainage of the abdomen.

(a) Post-operatively he vomits fresh blood.
   (i) State two possible causative factors. (1 mark)
   (ii) How would you treat these complications? (4 marks)

(b) The abdominal drain drains a clear fluid with a high amylase content.
   (i) State the significance of this finding. (1 mark)
   (ii) How would you identify the lesion? (2 marks)

(c) The abdominal drain drains bile instead.
- (i) State the probable lesion. (1 mark)
- (ii) How would you define the lesion? (1 mark)

Question 9

A 30-year-old man presents to the Accident and Emergency Department complaining of severe central abdominal pain and nausea of seven days' duration.

(a) In the absence of significant clinical findings a working diagnosis of acute non-specific abdominal pain was made.
  (i) What do you understand by this statement? (1 mark)
  (ii) Give examples of psychosomatic states that may be associated with this presentation. (2 marks)

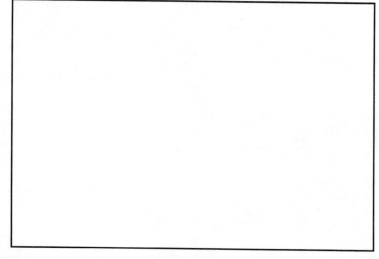

(b) Further enquiries revealed a history of alcoholism, with previous similar clinical presentations.
  (i) State the probable diagnosis and the investigations required to confirm this. (3 marks)
  (ii) Write a note on the principles of treatment. (4 marks)

CHAPTER 9: SMALL AND LARGE BOWEL

Question 1

A 79-year-old woman with a vague history of intermittent crampy lower abdominal pains underwent a colonoscopic examination. A cluster of polyps covering an area of 7 cm was seen in the descending colon.

(a) List three histological varieties of benign colonic polyps. (2 marks)

(b) How would you manage this condition? (5 marks)

(c) Outline the aetiology of this condition. (3 marks)

Question 2

An otherwise healthy 44-year-old woman gives a history of many years of increasing constipation that followed a difficult pregnancy and confinement. She is presently dependent on laxatives.

(a) List two causative factors. (2 marks)

(b) How would you assist this patient's symptoms? (3 marks)

(c) Outline your management. (5 marks)

Question 3

A 61-year-old man known to have diverticular disease on a previous colonoscopy is admitted as an emergency with crampy lower abdominal pains, fever, malaise and anorexia. Abdominal examination reveals mild peritonism in the lower left quadrant.

(a) State the probable cause of his symptoms. (2 marks)

(b) List two investigations that would support your diagnosis. (4 marks)

(c) Outline your management. (4 marks)

Question 4

A 3-month-old infant is referred to the Accident and Emergency Department with a three-day history of fretfulness and colic. He had vomited bile-stained fluid the previous day and passed blood-stained mucus per rectum.

(a) (i) State the likely diagnosis. (1 mark)
(ii) Write a note on the factors that may be associated with this condition. (2 marks)

(b) What would be the findings on abdominal examination? (3 marks)

(c) (i) State one investigation that is used both to confirm the diagnosis and to treat the condition. (1 mark)
(ii) How is this procedure performed? (3 marks)

Question 5

a 77-year-old woman is referred to the surgical clinic with a three-month history of alteration in bowel habit, with intermittent passage of loose motions containing mucus and blood.

(a) List the possible causes of her symptoms. (3 marks)

(b) If dietary and infective causes are excluded, outline the specific measures you would adopt to arrive at a diagnosis. (4 marks)

(c) If abdominal examination revealed hepatomegaly and ascites, state the further investigations you would request and the information obtained therefrom. (3 marks)

Question 6

A 59-year-old woman is admitted with a three-week history of progressively severe crampy lower abdominal pain and distension. She had not opened her bowels for the past nine days, felt nauseated and had vomited twice over the previous two days.

(a) (i) State your expected clinical findings. (2 marks)
(ii) What is your working diagnosis? (1 mark)

(b) (i) State one radiological investigation that would confirm your diagnosis. (1 mark)
(ii) List the findings. (2 marks)

(c) State your initial management of this patient. (4 marks)

Question 7

A 45-year-old, 70 kg man is admitted with symptoms of acute small bowel obstruction.

(a) List the findings on AXR which would confirm the diagnosis. (2 marks)

(b) (i) How would you assess the accompanying fluid and electrolyte derangement? (3 marks)
(ii) How would you treat it? (3 marks)

(c) If the obstruction is due to adhesions as a consequence of previous abdominal surgery, state your management. (2 marks)

Question 8

A 4-day-old neonate is seen in the Accident and Emergency Department with progressive abdominal distension and not passing meconium since birth.

(a) List the causes of large bowel obstruction in the newborn. (2 marks)

(b) Rectal examination on this patient was followed by a spontaneous passage of a large quantity of meconium.
(i) State the probable diagnosis. (1 mark)
(ii) Write a note on its pathogenesis. (3 marks)

(c) (i) State two investigations to confirm your diagnosis. (2 marks)
(ii) State the principles of surgical treatment. (2 marks)

Question 9

A neonate presents at birth with a defect in the abdominal wall, covered by a transparent sac containing loops of intestine. The umbilical cord was attached at its apex.

(a) (i) What is this condition called? (1 mark)
(ii) Write a note on the development of this anomaly. (3 marks)

(b) Write a note on the principles of treatment for this condition. (3 marks)

(c) List three malformations of the alimentary tract resulting in failure of canalisation of the lumen. (3 marks)

Question 10

A 43-year-old manual worker presented to the Accident and Emergency Department with a four-day history of fever and a painful, tender, fluctuant swelling immediately lateral to the anus.

(a) (i) State the probable diagnosis. (1 mark)
(ii) Write a note on the evolution of this lesion. (3 marks)

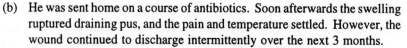

(b) He was sent home on a course of antibiotics. Soon afterwards the swelling ruptured draining pus, and the pain and temperature settled. However, the wound continued to discharge intermittently over the next 3 months.
(i) State the complication that had ensued. (1 mark)
(ii) How should his original lesion have been treated? (2 marks)
(iii) Write a note on the principles of treating the current complication. (3 marks)

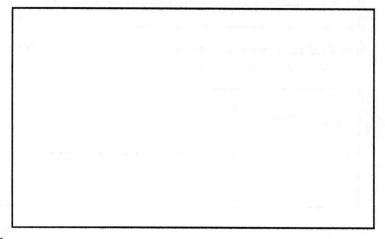

Question 11

A 35-year-old man is referred to the surgical clinic with a four-month history of painless rectal bleeding following defaecation.

(a) (i) How would you examine the ano-rectum to arrive at a diagnosis? (3 marks)
(ii) List three diseases of the colon that may present thus. (3 marks)

(b) The patient also complains of an intermittent fleshy protrusion at the anus.
(i) State the most likely cause. (1 mark)
(ii) List three procedures used in treating this condition. (3 marks)

Question 12

A 68-year-old woman presents with a six-week history of tenesmus and the passage of blood-stained mucus in her motions. Examination reveals an ulcerating lesion in the rectum.

(a) (i) How would you characterise the clinical features of this lesion? (3 marks)

(ii) State one investigation that is required to make a definitive diagnosis. (2 marks)

(b) A diagnosis of a rectal adenocarcinoma is made.

(i) State the most frequent site of blood-borne metastases. (1 mark)

(ii) What is your method of its detection? (1 mark)

(iii) Write a note on the surgical treatment of this lesion. (3 marks)

CHAPTER 10: UROLOGY

Question 1

A female neonate is found at birth to have a 5 cm defect in the lower abdominal wall through which urine was extravasating.

(a) State your diagnosis. (2 marks)

(b) List the structures that may be visible through the defect. (3 marks)

(c) State the associated anomalies that may be present. (2 marks)

(d) How would you manage this condition? (3 marks)

Question 2

A 2-year-old toddler is referred to the Surgical Clinic with a history from the parents of irritation and ballooning of the foreskin during micturition over a four-month period.

(a) (i) State the probable diagnosis. (2 marks)
(ii) How would you confirm your diagnosis? (2 marks)

(b) What are the complications of this condition? (3 marks)

(c) State your treatment. (3 marks)

Question 3

A 10-year-old Asian boy presents as an emergency in acute urinary retention. He gives a history of frequency with episodes of strangury, penile tip pain and haematuria over the past 18 months.

(a) State your working diagnosis. (2 marks)

(b) Outline your investigations. (4 marks)

(c) How would you treat this condition? (4 marks)

Question 4

A 29-year-old man is referred to the Surgical Clinic with a six-week history of an asymptomatic swelling in the right side of his scrotum.

(a) (i) State the structures that may be involved. (3 marks)
(ii) Describe how you would, by examination, localise the lesion. (2 marks)

(b) (i) List three testicular tumours found in young adults. (3 marks)
(ii) State the principles of treating testicular tumours. (2 marks)

Question 5

A middle-aged man is seen in the Surgical Clinic with an asymptomatic intermittent swelling in his right groin. He gives a 12-month history of nocturnal frequency and dribbling.

(a) State the nature of his groin swelling and examination findings that would support your diagnosis. (3 marks)

(b) State the probable cause of his urinary symptoms and discuss the relevant findings on examination. (3 marks)

(c) Discuss briefly the management of this patient. (4 marks)

Question 6

A 15-year-old boy presents to the Accident and Emergency department with sudden onset of severe pain in his left testicle two hours previously.

(a) (i) State the likely diagnosis. (1 mark)
(ii) State your findings in support of the diagnosis. (3 marks)

(b) Write a short note on your treatment. (3 marks)

(c) If the patient presented 48 hours after the onset of symptoms, how would this alter your management? (3 marks)

Question 7

A 70-year-old man complains of passing bubbles of gas in his urine. Six months previously he had undergone surgical removal of a colonic tumour, followed by radiotherapy to the region.

(a) (i) What is this symptom called? (1 mark)
    (ii) State two probable causes for this symptom. (2 marks)

(b) List the investigations that would confirm your diagnosis. (3 marks)

(c) List four other diseases that may produce this complication. (4 marks)

Question 8

A 75-year-old man is returned to the ward following transurethral prostatectomy. He complains of severe suprapubic pain and becomes hypotensive.

(a) State two surgical complications that would present thus. (4 marks)

(b) State two causes of prostatic enlargement that require prostatectomy. (2 marks)

(c) List the complications that may arise if symptoms of prostatism are left untreated. (4 marks)

Question 9

A 28-year-old man is referred to the urology clinic complaining of impotence.

(a) State three causes for this. (3 marks)

(b) Seminal fluid analysis suggested sterility. What criteria would this report be based on? (3 marks)

(c) (i) State a chronic infection that may produce sterility in this patient. (1 mark)
(ii) How would you confirm your diagnosis? (3 marks)

Question 10

A 35-year-old man in end-stage renal failure underwent cadaveric renal transplantation. Post-operatively he remains oliguric.

(a) List four possible causes for the oliguria. (2 marks)

(b) Write a note on the investigations you would perform to arrive at a diagnosis. (3 marks)

(c) (i) List the drugs used for immunosuppression following transplantation. (2 marks)
(ii) Write a note on the complications associated with their use. (3 marks)

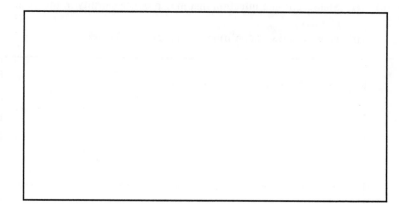

Question 11

A 28-year-old woman is referred to the urology clinic with a three-month history of severe intermittent unilateral loin pain radiating to the groin, accompanied by nausea and vomiting.

(a) (i) State your clinical diagnosis. (1 mark)
(ii) What immediate investigation would confirm your diagnosis at the bed side? (2 marks)

(b) Outline your management. (5 marks)

(c) List four predisposing causes. (2 marks)

Question 12

A 5-year-old boy presents to the paediatric surgical clinic with an incidental discovery of a left flank mass by his mother.

(a) (i) List four lesions of the kidney that may present thus. (2 marks)
(ii) State three imaging procedures used to arrive at a diagnosis. (3 marks)

(b) If these investigations reveal a malignant tumour of the left kidney.
(i) State three investigations required to determine the presence of distant metastases. (2 marks)
(ii) Outline the three modalities of treatment. (3 marks)

Question 13

A 34-year-old otherwise healthy male presents with progressive symptoms of straining to void, with poor urinary stream and dribbling. An indurated area was palpable in the line of the penile urethra.

(a) State the probable diagnosis and list the probable causes of this condition. (3 marks)

(b) State the complications of this lesion. (3 marks)

(c) Write a note on the principles of treatment. (4 marks)

Question 14

(a) Define stress incontinence of urine and discuss its causes in a 35-year-old woman. (3 marks)

(b) How would you investigate her symptoms? (3 marks)

(c) State the principles of treatment. (4 marks)

CHAPTER 11: VASCULAR SURGERY

Question 1

A 79-year-old man presents to the Accident and Emergency Department with a four-hour history of sudden onset of severe pain and numbness in his left leg extending up to his mid-thigh.

(a) State your working diagnosis and the predisposing vascular diseases. (3 marks)

(b) List the clinical findings in the limb supporting your diagnosis. (3 marks)

(c) Write a note on the treatment. (4 marks)

Question 2

A 68-year-old man complains of gradual onset of right calf claudication radiating up to his thigh on walking distances exceeding 75 yards.

(a) (i) State your likely diagnosis and the anatomic site(s) of his lesion. (2 marks)
(ii) Write a short note on the disease process causing his symptoms. (3 marks)

(b) Give four common risk factors in this disease. (2 marks)

(c) What measures would you advise him to adopt to alleviate his symptoms, to stop progression of the disease and improve his walking distance? (3 marks)

Question 3

A 59-year-old woman complains of rest pain in her left foot keeping her awake at night. She also had difficulty in walking.

(a) List the clinical findings that would lead to a working diagnosis. (4 marks)

(b) (i) Name one radiological investigation you would request to demonstrate the lesion. (1 mark)

(ii) Write a short note on how radiological procedures may be used to treat her symptoms. (2 marks)

(c) Discuss briefly the surgical options available to relieve her symptoms. (3 marks)

Question 4

A 68-year-old man underwent a femoral arteriogram and balloon angioplasty for an external iliac arterial stenosis.

(a) List the symptoms and clinical findings that would have led to this procedure. (3 marks)

(b) Soon afterwards he complained of severe pain in the limb, which had become blanched and pulseless.
  (i) State two likely causes for this complication. (2 marks)
  (ii) State your management. (3 marks)

(c) List the risk factors in the development of peripheral vascular disease. (2 marks)

Question 5

A 76-year-old man presents with a pulsatile swelling in his right groin three days after a coronary angioplasty at the site where the cardiac catheter was introduced.

(a) (i) State the most likely diagnosis. (1 mark)
(ii) State one non-invasive investigation for confirmation. (1 mark)
(iii) How would you treat this? (2 marks)

(b) The patient developed a cold, painful and pulseless lower limb immediately after the coronary angioplasty.
(i) State two probable causes. (2 marks)
(ii) How would you treat each of these complications? (4 marks)

Question 6

A 75-year-old man is referred to the surgical clinic with an incidental finding of a palpable, pulsatile and expansile upper abdominal mass of approximately 10 cm in diameter.

(a) (i) State the likely diagnosis. (1 mark)
(ii) Discuss the pathological changes that produced this lesion. (2 marks)

(b) State one non-invasive investigation you would request to identify the anatomical limits of the lesion. (1 mark)

(c) (i) Write short notes on the principles of surgical treatment of this patient. (3 marks)
(ii) Write short notes on the pre-operative preparation of the patient. (3 marks)

Question 7

A 64-year-old man is admitted to the Accident and Emergency Department complaining of severe back pain, radiating to the left loin accompanied by nausea and feeling faint. He was found to be hypotensive, with a rapid, thready pulse.

(a) (i) State your clinical diagnosis. (1 mark)
(ii) Outline your resuscitatory measures. (3 marks)

(b) State the surgical treatment for this condition. (1 mark)

(c) (i) If he were on long-term warfarin therapy for atrial fibrillation and his INR was found to be over 4.0, what would be your diagnosis? (2 marks)
(ii) State your specific treatment measures. (3 marks)

Question 8

A 70-year-old pensioner gives a history of dizzy spells over an eight-month period. More recently he experienced occasional blurring of vision, with transient loss of vision in his right eye.

(a) (i) Give the probable cause of his symptoms. (1 mark)
(ii) State the underlying factors that may be causative or associated with his disease. (2 marks)

(b) (i) Name one invasive investigation to confirm your diagnosis. (1 mark)
(ii) What information would you obtain therefrom? (2 marks)

(c) Write a note on your proposed treatment. (4 marks)

Question 9

A 50-year-old woman with a long history of progressively symptomatic lower limb varicosities bled profusely from a chronic leg ulcer. She presents to the Accident and Emergency Department with a tourniquet applied to control the haemorrhage.

(a) Write a note on the pathogenesis of the ulcer and the bleeding therefrom. (3 marks)

(b) Comment on the method used for haemostasis and state how you would control the bleeding. (3 marks)

(c) Discuss her management once haemostasis has been achieved. (4 marks)

Question 10

A middle-aged woman is seen in the surgical clinic with a long history of a painful ulcer over the medial aspect of her left ankle, with swelling of the foot. She also complained of long-standing varicose veins in that limb.

(a) (i) State the type of ulcer and its cause. (1 mark)
(ii) Comment on the characteristics of the lesion and the state of the surrounding skin. (2 marks)

(b) (i) Write a short note on the measures you would adopt to bring about the healing of the ulcer. (2 marks)
(ii) How would you prevent its recurrence? (1 mark)

(c) State two other types of chronic leg ulcers and discuss their pathophysiology. (4 marks)

Question 11

A 46-year-old woman who had undergone abdominal surgery five days previously develops pain and cramps in her left calf and lower thigh.

(a) Discuss the clinical findings you would elicit in order to arrive at a diagnosis. (3 marks)

(b) (i) State a diagnosis which carries potentially lethal complications. (1 mark)

(ii) Write a short note on the pathophysiology of this condition and its complications. (3 marks)

(c) Write a short note on the management of this patient. (3 marks)

Question 12

A 35-year-old woman who had been discharged from hospital two days previously, following abdominal surgery, develops sudden chest pain, with shortness of breath.

(a) (i) What is the most likely diagnosis? (1 mark)
(ii) State the two most important investigations to confirm your diagnosis. (2 marks)

(b) Discuss the treatment for this condition. (5 marks)

(c) List the preventive measures to avoid this complication. (2 marks)

SECTION II:
SAQ MODEL ANSWERS

CHAPTER 1: SURGICAL PHYSIOLOGY

Answer 1 **Marks**

(a) Conjugated bilirubin and alkaline phosphatase are markedly raised (normal: 7 umol.l and 0–306 units/l respectively); the raised amino and gamma-glutamyl transferases is suggestive of significant liver damage, which is reflected by a low serum albumin (normal: 2535 g/l) and decreased plama prothrombin index. 4

(b) Improve general nutritional status by high protein-calorie diet
Correct hypochromic anaemic
Vitamin K therapy to improve clotting profile 3

(c) Surgical bleeding (intra- and post-operative)
Poor wound healing
Post-operative liver failure 3

Comments

Patients in liver failure tolerate anaesthesia or surgery poorly. The Child's grading of liver failure in assessing pre-operative fitness is based on the serum bilirubin and albumin, presence of ascites, and neurological and nutritional status. Liver failure in the post-operative period requires monitoring and correction of blood sugar and electrolyte abnormalities, namely hypoglycaemia and hypernatraemia. Associated renal failure with hyperkalaemia and uraemia requires dialysis. Post-operative bleeding and infection are treated with the judicious use of blood products and parenteral antibiotics.

Answer 2

(a) FEV_1/FVC is 1.2/4/2 = 52% and indicates obstructive disease; following the administration of bronchodilators, a persisting low ratio suggests chronic obstructive airways disease (COAD) and an improved ratio suggests chronic asthma. 4

(b) Breathing exercises, postural physiotherapy to expectorate secretions Antibiotics to treat residual infection Oxygen therapy to improve gaseous exchange Stop smoking (if applicable)	**Marks** 3
(c) Mechanical ventilatory support with arterial blood gas (pulmonary artery wedge pressures if required) and chest radiographic monitoring with selective use of sedation, muscle relaxant and antibiotics in a high dependency or intensive therapy unit	3

Comment

The ratio FEV_1/FVC is normally 75%. A restrictive lung defect reduces both FEV_1 and FVC so that the ratio remains unaltered or may rise slightly, as in fibrosing alveolitis. An obstructive defect causes a relatively larger reduction in FEV1 so that the ratio falls, as in emphysema, chronic bronchitis and asthma. Pre-operative therapy is aimed at improving lung function to the optimum whilst recognizing the limits imposed by end-stage lung disease. Intensive care and ventilatory support following surgery must be available.

Answer 3

(a) (i) Hyperkalaemia and hypernatraemia Metabolic acidosis with uraemia	2
(ii) Gram-negative septicaemia Hypovolaemia	2
(b) Rehydration i.v. antibiotic therapy Fluid challenge with judicious use of loop diuretics Peri-operative haemofiltration if above measures fail to improve urinary output	4

Marks

Comment

Was this patient's renal function normal prior to his surgical illness? Evidence of a recent assessment of renal function may point to pre-existing renal disease (chronic nephritis) as the underlying cause of present renal failure. If previous renal function was normal and the present insult not treated promptly, the pre-renal cause would result in acute tubular necrosis. Overwhelming sepsis or disseminated intravascular coagulation result in renal failure and must be treated with haemodialysis or haemofiltration (peritoneal dialysis is contraindicated in view of abdominal sepsis and impending surgery). Haemodialysis results in a rapid correction of metabolic abnormalities, but also produces significant body fluid fluctuations. Haemofiltration produces less haemodynamic changes and is preferable in the acutely ill patient peri-operatively.

Answer 4

(a) (i) Thirst; skin turgor; BP (postural drop); serum urea and electrolyte measurement; urine output — 1

(ii) N/saline, 5% & 10%; dextrose 1.8% or 3.0% dextrose in normal saline; Hartmann's solution; KCl solution (amount in mmols to be carefully titrated against daily or twice daily serum levels) — 2

(iii) CVP monitoring; 3-hourly urea and electrolyte estimation; hourly urine output; daily Hb and PCV estimation; daily weighing of patient — 2

(b) (i) Hb, PCV, serum albumin, folate, B12, Fe; skinfold thickness by use of callipers — 2

(ii) Daily calorie and nitrogen requirements are calculated on the ideal weight for the patient's height and body build. Energy requirements vary from 1500 to 3000 kcal per day and are provided by administered carbohydrate 40% and lipid 60%. Daily nitrogen requirement is based on replacing existing protein depletion and ongoing breakdown in wear and tear. — 3

Comment **Marks**

Calories are provided by carbohydrate and fat. They should be in proportion to the nitrogen intake in the ratio of 150 kcal to 1 g of nitrogen. Administered nitrogen should not be used as an energy source, as it would perpetuate the state of negative nitrogen balance. The patient receiving 2000 kcal would require 13 g of nitrogen daily. Vitamins and trace elements are essential as dietary supplements for normal metabolic function and must be included in feeding regimes.

Answer 5

(a) (i) Metabolic (hypokalaemic, hyponatraemic, hypochloraemic) alkalosis 1

(ii) The fluid regime did little to correct the Na^+ and K^+ ion loss in vomit and gastric aspirate 3

(b) Gastric outlet obstruction leads to loss of water, Na^+, K^+ and H^+ ions. Anti-diuretic hormone production is stimulated by the hypothalamus. This results in renal tubular resorption of Na^+ and K^+ ions at the expense of H^+ ions, which produces an acid urine, thereby exacerbating the metabolic alkalosis 6

Comment

The inappropriate production of acid urine in metabolic alkalosis is due to renal tubular response to dehydration and low serum [Na^+] by resorption of Na^+ and excretion of H^+ and K^+ in order to maintain trans-cellular ionic equilibrium. Counteractive measures should replace Na^+ and K^+ along with water by infusion with 0.9% (normal) saline with KCl supplementation. This would gradually reverse the alkalosis with a rise in urinary pH over the ensuing days.

Answer 6

(a) (i) Surgical trauma stimulates anti-diuretic hormone production with retention of salt and water 2

(ii) He would require no electrolyte supplements. Water requirements would be less than the normal daily

Marks

requirement of 2–3 litres per day and would be determined by the CVP reading. Five per cent dextrose is transfused to keep the CVP at approximately 2–6 cm of water 2

(b) (i) A normal CVP and BP would ensure good renal perfusion. A post-renal cause must be excluded by ensuring patency of catheter drainage. A low CVP is treated by volume replacement and a persistent low BP with pressure support using IV dopamine or dobutamine. The rate of elevation of serum urea and creatinine would indicate the extent of renal malfunction: this is nearly always due to acute tubular necrosis due to prolonged hypotension or a coagulopathy. A renal isotope scan would reveal the functional state of each kidney 4

(ii) Renal failure requires haemofiltration or haemodialysis to lower the urea and creatinine and to maintain electrolyte balance 2

Comment

Acute tubular necrosis is a sequela of major trauma, surgical or otherwise, where there is significant blood loss resulting in renal ischaemia. Cross-clamping the aorta in the vicinity of the renal arteries may also produce a fall in renal perfusion. Large volume transfusion with stored blood in the perioperative period may produce a coagulopathy, causing acute intravascular coagulation which may lead to renal damage and failure. Acute tubular necrosis usually recovers, and during recovery there is a diuresis, when large quantities of fluid and electrolytes are lost. Careful monitoring and replacement is therefore essential until complete renal function returns.

Answer 7

(a) (i) Pyrexial reactions are due to allergens and Gram-negative endotoxins in the donor blood. The skin rash is produced by agglutination of the donor cells in the

Marks

skin capillaries due to incompatibility with the recipient serum 2

(ii) Stop the transfusion immediately; set up a crystalloid infusion to produce a diuresis. Administer an antihistamine and an antipyretic agent as required 2

(b) (i) Acute liver failure and hepatic coma are rare complications and are precipitated by underlying liver disease. Some clotting factors are inactivated in stored blood, and a coagulopathy manifesting as acute intravascular coagulation leads to a bleeding diathesis in the post-operative period 2

(ii) In stored blood the plasma K^+ ions rise to 30–40 mmol/l and produce hyperkalaemia in the recipient. This may be treated by insulin administration with a covering dextrose infusion or by the ingestion of ion-exchange resin (calcium resonium). Citrated blood lowers the plasma Ca^{++} ion concentration in the recipient and it is treated by administration of calcium gluconate or calcium chloride 4

Comment

The signs of a mismatched blood transfusion include fever, chills, breathlessness, pain in the flanks and chest. These may be followed by hypotension, haemorrhagic phenomena and haemoglobinaemia. The last signals renal damage, which is exacerbated by hypotension and acidosis. The initial reactions occur during the first 30 minutes of the transfusion, and this period must be closely monitored when setting up a blood transfusion.

Answer 8

(a) (i) Lowered platelet count
Lowered vitamin K levels
Raise prothrombin and partial thromboplastin times 2

(ii) Lowered Hb
Lowered WBC count (viz. CD4 cells)

			Marks
		Lowered platelet count Lowered serum albumin (hypoproteinaemia) Lowered immunoglobulins	3
(b)	(i)	Plastic apron and non-porous sterile gowns Visors or goggles Double gloving Theatre footwear or shoe covers	2
	(ii)	Avoid passing instruments 'hand-to-hand' Avoid 'sharps' by using cutting diathermy or a harmonic scalpel for sharp dissection Scissors with bevelled ends Blunt needles Metal or plastic clips for haemostasis and wound closure	3

Comment

Patients with HIV infection have an increased risk of primary and secondary haemorrhage and post-surgical bacterial infection. Wound healing is also delayed due to hypoproteinaemia from cachexia. The grave dangers of accidental inoculation with tissue fluids from HIV patients during operations should ensure familiarity with safety measures formulated to protect theatre personnel.

Answer 9

(a)	(i)	Metabolic acidosis	1
	(ii)	Ketoacidosis Lactic acidosis Renal failure	2
(b)	(i)	Plasma glucose U&E and creatinine	3
	(ii)	IV normal saline or Hartmann's solution IV K^+ infusion guided by U&E estimation IV insulin on a sliding scale IV antibiotics – flucloxacillin (or cefuroxime) and metronidazole	

Measure: **Marks**
4-hourly ABG
4-hourly U&E
2-hourly serum K^+ 4

Comment

A variety of organic acids are produced during metabolic activity and their effects are counteracted by expelling CO_2 in the lungs and excreting an acid urine. During metabolic or surgical illness the body is unable to counter the acid load produced, leading to metabolic acidosis. Determination of the base excess and HCO_3^- in arterial blood enables effective countermeasures. In addition to the measures stated, 4.8% $NaHCO_3$ IV infusion is indicated if the acidosis is intractable or is causing cardiac arrhythmias, confusion or drowsiness. 2

Answer 10

(a) (i) He has been unable to eat or drink properly due to difficulty in swallowing 1

(ii) Moderate to severe protein–calorie (energy) malnutrition 1

(iii) Visible muscle wasting with reduced muscle strength. Lax subcutaneous tissue from loss of fat deposits as shown by skinfold thickness 2

(b) (i) By enteral feeding through a fine-bore nasogastric tube or by total parenteral nutrition. By either route 1.5–2.5 litres of fluid containing 2000–2500 kcal and 1.5 g of protein per kg body weight is infused every 24 hours 3

(ii) Daily measurements of body weight
Input and output fluid charts
Serum U&Es, albumin, glucose and urinary glucose
Twice-weekly measurements of Hb, Ca^{++}, Mg^{++}, triglycerides, urinary creatinine, Na^+ and K^+ 3

Comment

Nutrient solutions, whether enteral or parenteral, must be administered in moderate increments during the first 48 hours to avoid hyperosmolarity of the body fluids and to give time for pancreatic adaptation. Extraneous insulin may be required to maintain the blood sugar within normal limits. Vitamins and trace elements are added daily. Skin callipers are used in some centres to quantify subcutaneous fat loss. A feeding gastrostomy or jejunostomy should be avoided if the patient is to undergo surgery for his stricture.

CHAPTER 2: TRAUMA AND BURNS

Answer 1 **Marks**

(a) Glasgow coma scale (see ***Comment***) 2

(b) Blood pressure, pulse and respiration
Pupillary sizes and reflexes
Eye movements (extrinsic muscles)
Abdominal reflexes; Cremasteric reflex
Limbs: Tone
Power, clonus
Reflexes (triceps, biceps, brachioradialis, knee jerk, ankle jerk, plantar reflex) 3

(c) (i) Extra(epi)dural
Subdural
Subarachnoid
Intracerebral
CT/MRI Head scan 2

(ii) Protect the airway
Exclude injury to cervical spine
Record blood pressure and pulse, with head injury observations ¼-hourly
Daily arterial blood gases
FBC and U&E
Intracranial pressure monitoring
Mannitol infusion preoperatively
Surgical evacuation of haematoma with placement of intra-cranial pressure monitoring device
Postoperative antibiotic therapy 3

Comment

Glasgow coma scale:		Score
	spontaneous	4/5
	to speech	3/4
Eyes open	to pain	2
	none	1

			Marks
Verbal response	orientated	5	
	confused	4	
	inappropriate	3	
	incomprehensible	2	
	none	1	
Motor response	obeys commands	5	
	localizes pain	4	
	flexion to pain	3	
	extension to pain	2	
	none	1	
Best total score		14/15	

In all forms of intra-cranial bleeding, the time between injury and decompression is a major determinant of outcome. The onus should, therefore, be on rapid evacuation to a neurosurgical centre for appropriate management.

Recovery from surgical evacuation of intracranial haematoma is slow and unpredictable. The multidisciplinary rehabilitation team should include neurosurgical, psychiatric, speech and physiotherapy, and social and community services.

Answer 2

(a) Clinically assess airway patency and air exchange, viz oropharynx for foreign body or mucus plug obstruction, respiratory movements. Monitor pulse and BP. Establish peripheral and central venous access for CVP, ABG and pulmonary arterial wedge pressure measurements; FBC and U&E. Administer O_2 by face mask. Record ECG — 3

(b) Tension/open pneumothorax (including flail chest)
Massive haemothorax
Cardiac tamponade — 2

(c) (i) Promptly close defect in chest wall with sterile occlusive dressings large enough to overlap wound edges and tape securely on three sides to provide a flutter valve effect. Site a chest drain remote from the wound. Close the wound surgically when the patient's condition is stable — 2

Marks

(ii) Decide drain site on CXR, usually at 5th intercostal space on anterior or mid-axillary line. Infiltrate area with lignocaine (1 or 2%) or bupivacaine (0.5%). Make skin incision, enter pleural cavity by blunt dissection and introduce tube drain on introducer into pleural cavity. Connect drain to under-water seal. Secure drain and close wound around it with non-absorbable sutures 3

Comment

Flail chest occurs when a segment of the chest wall becomes detached from the rib cage. It leads to 'paradoxical breathing' but may be initially masked due to splinting of the chest wall from pain. Mechanical ventilation is usually indicated.

Massive haemothorax results from a rapid loss of 1–2 litres of blood into the pleural cavity and must be suspected when shock is associated with absent breath sounds and dullness to percussion on that side. Initial management is by simultaneous restoration of blood volume and decompression of the pleural cavity. Continued blood loss (>200 ml/hr) may require thoracotomy.

Cardiac tamponade presents as paradoxical elevation of the JVP on inspiration, fall in arterial pulse pressure and muffled heart sounds (Beck's triad). Pericardiocentesis is indicated when response to resuscitation is poor and the diagnosis suspected. Tracings on a cardiac monitor may reveal injury patterns which along with a positive pericardiocentesis would require thoracotomy and inspection of the heart.

Answer 3

(a) (i) Right-sided tension pneumothorax
Right haemothorax 2

(ii) Tracheal shift to left
Hyper-resonant or dull to percussion, with diminished or absent breath sounds in the right chest
Evidence of injury to chest wall on gently springing the rib cage 2

Marks

(b) (i) ABG 1

(ii) Postero-anterior and lateral chest X-ray 1

(c) Pulmonary contusion
Myocardial contusion
Aortic disruption
Diaphragmatic rupture
Tracheo-bronchial disruption
Oesophageal disruption 4

Comment

Pulmonary and myocardial contusions are the most common potentially lethal chest injuries. In the former, respiratory failure may be subtle and develop over time, and in the latter the diagnosis is made by abnormalities on the ECG. Traumatic aortic rupture is a cause of sudden death; potential survivors tend to have a laceration near the ligamentum anteriosum of the aorta, continuity being maintained by an intact adventitial layer. Many survivors die in hospital if the injury is unrecognised. A cardinal radiological sign is a widened mediastinum, caused by the haematoma surrounding the aorta. Blunt traumatic disruption to the tracheo-bronchial tree, oesophagus and diaphragm may all present late, and operative repair with drainage is life-saving. Unlike immediately life-threatening conditions these injuries may not be obvious on initial examination, and timely diagnosis is often based on a high index of clinical suspicion.

Answer 4

(a) (i) Liver, spleen, pancreas, duodenum, diaphragm, kidneys, urinary bladder 2

(ii) Ultrasound scan or CT of abdomen 1

(b) (i) Quarter-hourly BP, pulse and respiration
Check urine for blood
Half-hourly urine output; catheterize if required
FBC, ABG, CXR, AXR 2

Marks

(ii) Peripheral and central venous access for volume replacement and CVP monitoring. Intubation and mechanical ventilation for respiratory decompensation 2

(c) Developing signs of peritonism and an increase in abdominal girth signify intraperitoneal haemorrhage or rupture of a hollow viscus. Imaging of the abdomen or a diagnostic peritoneal lavage would detect bleeding and/or visceral injuries before the onset of lethal complications (oligaemia and/or toxic shock). 3

Comment

Unrecognised abdominal injury remains a frequent cause of preventable death after trauma. Peritoneal signs are often overshadowed by pain from associated injuries. Diagnostic peritoneal lavage under local anaesthetic can alter subsequent physical signs but does reveal the presence of intraperitoneal bleeding or bowel contents. A laparoscopic examination under a general anaesthetic may be useful when a significant visceral injury is suspected. It will confirm the diagnosis and determine the extent of the injury and the need for surgery.

Answer 5

(a) Resuscitation order:
Ensure airway patency and adequate ventilation by administering supplementary oxygen; intubate and ventilate manually if necessary
Immobilise cervical spine and place patient on a long spine board
Restore circulatory blood volume by crystalloids, plasma expanders and colloids as necessary with pulse, BP and JVP monitoring
Commence head injury observations
Alleviate pain with narcotic analgesics
Perform careful and thorough physical examination 5

(b) Counter hypothermia, administer O_2 and support ventilation, set up i.v. infusion and maintain normal b lood pressure
Maintain constant verbal and tactile communication and reassure the conscious patient

Marks

Treat life- and limb-threatening emergencies as facilities permit (e.g. close open chest would with occlusive dressing, control external haemorrhage with pressure dressing, re-align displaced limb fractures) 3

(c) 1 anaesthetist
1 trauma surgeon
1 trauma nurse
1 paramedic
1 pilot
(Helicopter capacity rarely exceeds 6 persons, including the patient and equipment) 2

Comment

Resuscitation is best carried out in the ambulance, except in respiratory or cardiac arrest, when intubation and external cardiac massage are performed at the roadside. When immediate extraction of the victim from the wreckage is not possible, life support is continued and consideration given to the need for on-site amputation of a severely injured trapped limb.

Answer 6

(a) Cervical spine: fracture of vertebral arches or bodies with/without dislocation. Cervical cord: concussion, incomplete lesion, hemisection, transection 2

(b) Skin bruising on the lateral and/or posterior aspects of the neck; neck muscle spasm 1

Attempt to elicit passive movement! 1

(c) (i) Reduction and stabilisation of fracture by cervical traction or internal fixation in selected patients 2

(ii) Care of nutritional requirements and prevention of catabolic state
Prevention and treatment of respiratory and/or urinary infections
Skin care to prevent pressure sores
Physiotherapy to prevent joint contractures 4

Comment **Marks**

Patients with suspected spinal injuries must be assessed following immbolization on a long spine board with a semi-rigid collar and neck support. Cervical spine injuries are caused by flexion, rotation, compression and hyperextension. Indication for surgery is progression of neurological deficit despite reduction and external stabilisation. Spinal fusion avoids prolonged bed rest with its associated morbidity.

Answer 7

(a) (i) Use 'Rule of Nines' (modified for infants and toddlers)
Affected area: approximately 18% 1

(ii) Verbal reassurance
Pain relief and sedation
Tetanus prophylaxis
Wound toilet: the burn surface is either left exposed or covered with dressing impregnated with silver nitrate or an antibiotic in an oil or water base
Prophylactic antibiotic therapy for 5–10 days 4

(b) (i) Partial thickness injury appears moist, red and blistered, with preservation of pain sensation. Full-thickness injury is usually white or brown, dry, firm and insensitive to touch 2

(ii) Body weight in kg x % of burned surface = amount of fluid in ml is the amount required in the first four hours. Monitor haematocrit and hourly urine output and give same amount over next four hours. Provided the clinical state is stable, give the same amount over the next 16 hours. (Approximately half colloid and half crystalloid solutions) 3

Comment

The child may develop paralytic ileus and for the first 6–8 hours the oral intake should be restricted to 50 ml of water per hour and thereafter gradually increased to half-strength milk, followed by a liquid diet.

Marks

Immediate tangential excision of the burn with split-skin grafting reduces fluid and protein loss, prevents infection and accelerates healing.

Answer 8

(a) Smoke inhalation injury (respiratory tract burns) 1

Humidified oxygen by face mask
Ambu-bag ventilation if required
Calm patient with reassurance
Mild sedation if necessary 2

(b) (i) Laryngeal oedema and/or oedema of the lower respiratory tract with bronchospasm 2

(ii) Endotracheal intubation with assisted ventilation. Tracheostomy if prolonged mechanical ventilation is required 2

(iii) Relieve bronchospasm with bronchodilators and steroids (as required). Positive pressure ventilation if arterial blood gases deteriorate. Prophylactic systemic antibiotic cover. Intravenous crystalloid administration to maintain hydration and renal function 3

Comment

Inability to intubate orally requires emergency cricothyroidotomy and tracheal intubation as severe respiratory burns lead rapidly to respiratory failure and death. Lesser degrees of bronchial and alveolar damage lead to the 'shock lung syndrome', with increased airway resistance, raised pulmonary arterial wedge pressure and right ventricular strain. Cardio-pulmonary support in an intensive therapy unit until lung function recovers.

Answer 9

(a) (i) Apply semi-rigid cervical collar
Support spine during lifting and log rolling
Strap patient in a neutral position on a long spine board

Marks

fer to hospital with sand bags to support head, neck and shoulders 2

(ii) A lateral X-ray showing the base of the skull, all seven cervical vertebrae and the first thoracic vertebra
An antero-posterior neck X-ray to include an open mouth odontoid view
An antero-posterior view of the dorsal spine 2

(b) (i) Flaccid areflexia, especially with a flaccid rectal sphincter
Diaphragmatic breathing
Passive flexion but not extension at the elbow
Grimaces to painful stimuli above but not below the clavicle
Hypotension with bradycardia
Priapism (an uncommon but characteristic sign) 3

(c) Neurogenic shock results from injury to descending sympathetic pathways in the spinal cord, with loss of vasomotor tone and sympathetic innervation to the heart. The former causes intravascular pooling of blood and consequent hypotension, and the latter causes inability to increase the heart rate and produces bradycardia. The blood pressure, therefore, cannot be restored by fluid infusion alone, and the judicious use of vasopressor agents may be required 3

Comment

Three tracts are readily assessed clinically in evaluating a spinal cord injury. The corticospinal tract controls motor power on the same side and is tested by voluntary muscle contractions or involuntary response to painful stimuli. The spinothalamic tract transmits pain and temperature sensations to the opposite side and is tested by pinch or pin prick. The posterior columns carry proprioceptive impulses from the same side and are tested by position sense of the fingers and toes or tuning fork vibrations. A complete spinal cord lesion abolishes distal neurological function and prognosis for recovery is poor. Incomplete spinal cord lesions are compatible with recovery, and a careful examination to determine the presence of any sensory or motor function is, therefore, essential.

Answer 10 **Marks**

(a) (i) Primary survey detects tracheal deviation and rib injury (by gently springing the rib cage) and the presence of:

Central cyanosis
Paradoxical breathing
Surgical emphysema
Abdominal skin bruising or tenderness
CXR 2

(ii) Plain A–P view of the pelvis, ultrasound scan and/or CT of abdomen and pelvis and/or diagnostic peritoneal lavage or laparoscopic examination
Catheterize and examine urine for blood 2

(iii) Gentle palpation for a fracture and/or dislocation
Antero-posterior and lateral X-rays of the hip, femur, knee, tibia, fibula and ankle 2

(b) Establish two large-calibre i.v. peripheral lines
Establish a central venous line for CVP monitoring
Send blood for FBC, ABG, grouping and emergency cross-match
Transfuse with crystalloid solution (e.g. Ringer lactate) and a plasma volume expander (e.g. Haemacel) until whole blood is available to restore blood volume 4

Comment

The pulse and BP are monitored quarter-hourly, though these are poor measures of tissue perfusion. A pulse oximeter measures the saturation of haemoglobin colorimetrically (it is not a measure of partial pressure of oxygen); a small sensor is clipped onto the finger, toe or earlobe and displays the pulse rate and oxygen concentration continuously and reflects the respiratory and circulatory status.

Hypovolaemic shock may not respond to fluid therapy alone. Once the circulatory blood volume has been replaced and if tissue perfusion has not recovered due to peripheral vascular shutdown, judicious use of steroids and pressor agents to maintain renal and cerebral perfusion may be appropriate in an intensive care setting.

Answer 11 **Marks**

(a) Extent: Chest and abdomen make up 18% and each arm 7% of total body surface area ('Rule of Nines' modified for infants and toddlers)
Depth: Partial-thickness (epidermal) scald blanches on pressure, is pink and may blister, and is painful to pinprick
Full-thickness scald does not blanch, is pale or dull brown, and is devoid of pain (negative pinprick) 3

(b) Scalds exceeding 10% of body surface or a full-thickness scald exceeding $2.5cm^2$
Unrelated but significant underlying illness, e.g. diabetes, heart disease or epilepsy
Injury suspected of being non-accidental
Poor home circumstances 3

(c) Open method: expose surface moistened with antibacterial agents, in an environment of sterile ambient air
Closed method: Cover area with sterile occlusive non-adherent dressings impregnated with antibacterial agents. These are chlorhexidine-impregnated tulle gras, has anti-staphylococcal action; 1% sulphadiazine cream, has anti Gram-negative action (e.g. *Pseudomonas*, *Klebsiella*, *E. coli*); 10% sulphamylon cream, has same spectrum as above but penetrates avascular tissue; 0.5% silver nitrate solution soaked in cotton gauze, is bacteriostatic 4

Comment

Details of the circumstances of the injury must be obtained from an accompanying adult. The temperature of the liquid, whether clothing was worn, the exposure time, and if the surface was cooled with tap water or cold milk soon afterwards, are important in assessing wound depth and prognosis. The time interval between scalding and presentation, if more than six hours, is likely to result in an infection. Tetanus prophylaxis or immunisation is administered on presentation; pain relief, sedation and oral intake following IV hydration is monitored in the ensuing days. Bacterial colonization of the injured surface is usually complete in 24–48 hours. This may manifest as a local infection or may result in systemic spread, with fever and rigors. Prophylactic antibiotic therapy is therefore indicated in scalds exceeding 10% of the surface. **Marks**

Answer 12

(a) Airway patency and respiratory function (A+B)
Cardiac function by recording the pulse, BP and electrical activity on a cardiac monitor (C)
Level of consciousness: GCS score chart (D) 3

(b) Full-thickness burn wounds at entry and exit sites with variable underlying tissue destruction and damage to intervening tissue, viz subcutaneous fat and muscle 3

(c) Heart: ectopic rhythms, arrhythmias, ventricular fibrillation leading to cardiac arrest
Kidneys: acute renal failure due to (i) reduced perfusion during the shock phase, (ii) released haemoglobin red cells and damaged muscle
Muscle: tetanic contractions leading to joint and soft tissue injuries
Brain: convulsions leading to cerebral oedema
Peripheral nerves: conduction defects 4

Comment

The ABCDE of primary assessment is followed. Immediate cardiopulmonary resuscitation is commenced in ventricular arrhythmias. ECG monitoring and cardiac enzyme estimations detect injury to the heart muscle. Tissue destruction in high voltage electrical injuries is extensive and may progress as initially viable tissue necroses, due to vascular thrombosis and capillary damage. In addition to wound debridement, excision of dead or poorly viable muscle is required to prevent myoglobinuria and gas gangrene. Wounds must be left open, as progressive muscle necrosis is likely and may require further debridement. Early fasciotomy may be required if limb swelling progresses, to preserve its blood supply. Sustained diuresis is required to prevent renal failure from the breakdown products of muscle damage.

Answer 13 **Marks**

(a) The loss of serous fluid from the burned surface is replaced by plasma in the form of plasma protein fraction (PPF) or fresh frozen plasma (FFP) in four-hourly alliquots calculated as follows:

% burn area x patient's body weight x ½ (in ml)

This initial guide is modified by the clinical, haematological and biochemical profiles during the 24-hour period 3

(b) Wound debridement and toilet
Keep wound surface warm and moist with open or closed methods
Take wound culture swabs from multiple sites daily
Cover burned area early by homografts or heterografts which are renewed in the ward until the entire area is autografted from the patient's own donor sites
Correct dehydration, hypoproteinaemia and anaemia
Ensure adequate oral nutritional intake 4

(c) Ensure adequate pain relief with IV opiates and optimal fluid and electrolyte balance
The patient may only have a few hours of clarity of thought left before lapsing into confusion or coma. Therefore, explain the probable outcome and prognosis and the therapeutic options gently and dispassionately so that the patient's wishes on further management may be adhered to. Maximise time spent with loved ones and relatives with ready access to counsellor or priest. Seclude the patient from extraneous ward activity. 3

Comment

The extent of the burn injury is estimated by the 'Rule of Nines'. The depth of the burn should be mapped out and may be broadly divided into superficial (partial thickness) or deep (full thickness). The former involves the epidermis and superficial layers of the dermis and, in the latter, the epidermis and dermis are destroyed with a variable extent of underlying tissue. A third type

Marks

that is occasionally seen is the deep dermal burn where some of the germinal layers are spared but healing is poor and protracted, with wound contracture and scarring. Flame burns are nearly always deep, and the burn surface is debrided by tangential excision and covered by 'split skin' grafts taken from the patient's own donor sites. However, when the burn area is larger than the available donor sites, banked cadaver or pig skin may be used as temporary dressings until the area is grafted in stages by the patient's own skin. The former must be renewed every few days to prevent adherence and bleeding. There is no reliable evidence that using such 'other skin' dressings is superior to conventional antiseptic-impregnated, non-adherent gauze. Survival following a burn injury is dependent on the patient's age, the burn area and depth. In the very young, the very old and the chronically ill, the morbidity is high, from complications of the burn injury.

Answer 14

(a) Patient 2
Patient 1
Patient 4
Patient 3
Patient 5 — 3

(b) Patient 2: severe head injury; in acute respiratory distress due to airway compromise; also has major limb fractures; requires urgent airway control (A) and ventilatory support (B), volume replacement (C) and neurological assessment (D)

Patient 1: probable crush injury to the chest with major limb fractures; requires airway control (A) and ventilatory support (B) and volume replacement (C)

Patient 4: probable cervical spine injury with cord compression/damage; requires urgent stabilization on a spine board (A) and neurological assessment (D)

Marks

Patient 3: uterine trauma with probable fetal distress, requires fetal monitoring and sedation

Patient 5: bilateral ankle fractures and probable fracture/dislocation of the right hip 7

Comment

In the severely injured patient the 'golden hour' following injury is when resuscitatory measures have far-reaching effects on outcome and morbidity. Severe injuries kill or maim in specific reproducible timeframes. Thus ABCD or resuscitation prioritizes the assessment and resuscitation of organ systems in the following order:

- A Airway with Cervical spine control
- B Breathing
- C Circulation
- D Disability (neurological).

Answer 15

(a) Patient 2
Patient 4
Patient 3
Patient 5
Patient 1 3

(b) Patient 2: external haemorrhage; ? internal injuries/bleeding; requires urgent volume replacement (C), cervical spine control (A) and head injury assessment (D)

Patient 4: flail segment right ribcage with probable tension pneumothorax and lung collapse; probable crush injury to the abdomen; requires urgent airway control (A) and ventilatory support (B) and volume replacement (C)

Patient 3: crush injuries and fractures of both lower limbs; will be hypovolaemic; requires pain relief, volume replacement and assessment of lower limb perfusion (C); renal function requires close monitoring

Marks

Patient 5: severe psychological trauma; appears not be have suffered physical injury; requires full injury survey and sedation

Patient 1: asphyxiated (A, B) with cerebral anoxia (D) and hypovolaemia (C) with cardiac failure; unlikely to respond to resuscitation 7

Comment

Active resuscitation of patients with a low priority alongside those of a higher priority is dependent on the clinical resources available. However, in patients with a poor expectation of survival, active measures may only be abandoned following a negative or unsustainable physiological response to resuscitation. The time lapse between the injury and the commencement of resuscitation largely determines the outcome of severe injuries. This is particularly true of victims of natural disasterss when long delays may be inevitable, where communication and transport systems are disrupted and rescue efforts require the mobilization of rescue teams with logistic support.

Answer 16

(a) Patient 5
Patient 2
Patient 1
Patient 4
Patient 3 3

(b) Patient 5: despite the absence of external burns, smoke inhalation has compromised alveolar gaseous exchange resulting in cerebral hypoxia; requires urgent airway control (A) and assisted ventilation with oxygen therapy (B) to improve cerebral oxygenation (D) and for the management of the 'shock lung syndrome'

Patient 2: fracture of the shoulder girdle with a suspected cervical spine injury; requires urgent spinal immobilization (A) and pain relief

Marks

Patient 1: significant surface burn area, inhalation injury and blood loss from the scalp laceration; requires urgent ventilatory support and oxygen therapy (B), volume replacement (C) and pain control

Patient 4: non-life-threatening injuries requiring pain control, psychological support and volume replacement

Patient 3: 65% surface burns and inhalation injury with cerebral hypoxia at the age of 72 suggests a poor prognostic outcome despite intensive therapy 7

Comment

Clinical evidence of an inhalation injury from heat or fumes can be a history of explosion or confinement in a burning environment, facial burns, singing of eyebrows or nasal vibrissae, hoarseness or coughing up of carbonaceous sputum, acutely inflamed oropharynx and impaired cerebration. Carbon monoxide poisoining must be assumed in these patients and assisted ventilation and oxygen therapy instituted urgently.

Answer 17

(a) All medical teams on call
All laboratory personnel on call
Head of nursing services
Chief pharmacist
Medical Director
Chief Administrator (Chief Executive Officer)
Switchboard operator on duty would summon the above when instructed to put the disaster plan into action 3

(b) Accident and Emergency Department foyer as the reception area for all casualties
Accident and Emergency Department as the red coded area
Day Surgery unit as the yellow coded area
Outpatient Department as the blue coded area
Hospital foyer as the reception area for relatives and the media 3

(c) Casualties are received and triaged into three colour-coded categories, as follows: **Marks**

- Red — critcally injured and those requiring urgent resuscitation
- Yellow — severe and moderately severe non-life-threatening injuries
- Blue — minor injuries, i.e. the 'walking wounded' and those with post-traumatic stress symptoms 4

Comment

A major incident calls for the immediate implementation of the emergency disaster plan. This involves the immediate mobilization of pre-determined hospital personnel (including those not on duty at the time) to the designated reception and treatment areas; a senior clinician is nominated to co-ordinate operations in each area. The group allocated to the reception area assesses and triages patients to the treatment areas coded red, yellow and blue. The transfer of patients requiring specialized care to regional centres following stabilization is co-ordinated by a senior clinician. Beds are to be made available for those requiring admission and may involve the transfer of convalescent inpatients to other hospitals. A senior manager arranges technical and catering services to be made available to patients and staff.

CHAPTER 3: ORTHOPAEDICS

Answer 1 **Marks**

(a) Plain radiology of the femur and knee joint
Open biopsy of the lesion 2

(b) Ewing's sarcoma
Chondroblastoma
Osteosarcoma 3

(c) Counselling the child and parents/carers regarding treatment, reconstructive surgery or prosthetic fitting
Pre-operative radiotherapy
Radical surgery with complete tumour resection
Limb reconstruction or prosthetic fitting
Adjuvant chemotherapy 5

Comment

Osteosarcoma and chondroblastoma rarely present with consitutional symptoms, whereas Ewing's sarcoma, which arises in the diaphysis or metphysis of long bones, may give rise to malaise, pyrexia and a raised ESR, simulating osteomyelitis. Radiological appearances of these tumours show new bone formation with 'sun ray' spicules of new bone or subperiosteal new bone formation alongside areas of bone destruction. Radiotherapy and/or chemotherapy may precede surgery to control metastatic spread and to produce tumour regression. Radical surgery, the mainstay of treatment, may be accompanied by reconstruction of the bone and the adjacent joint with prosthetic implants or bone allografts to restore function and appearance.

Answer 2

(a) Lumbar intervertebral disc prolapse/protrusion, traumatic or degenerative in origin; rupture of the fibrous covering of disc leads to herniation of the disc pulp into the spinal canal, causing compression of the nerve roots that issue from the intervertebral foramina above and below the prolapsed disc' spinal canal tumours and metastatic tumour deposits are rare causes of nerve root irritation 3

Marks

(b) Pain and/or sensory loss in (i) groin suggests first lumbar root; (ii) front of mid or lower thigh with quadriceps muscle weakness and diminished knee jerk suggests second and third lumbar roots; (iii) back or side of thigh, lateral aspect of leg and dorsum of foot with quadriceps and anterior tibial muscle weakness and diminished knee jerk suggests fourth and fifth lumbar roots; (iv) sensory loss over dorsum of foot and specific weakness on dorsiflexion of the great toe suggests fifth root; (v) loss of sensation in sole of foot, weakness on plantar flexion and an absent knee jerk suggests first sacral root compression 3

(c) Initial measures are complete bedrest, analgesia and muscle relaxants; if symptoms do not settle or there is neurological deterioration or involvement of sphincter function, spinal CT or MRI scan may delineate the site of cord/root compression requiring surgical decompression; this usually consists of an open laminectomy, removing the debris in the intervertebral disc space and freeing the nerve roots; spinal fusion may be required to stabilize the spine; minimally invasive surgery may be feasible for root decompression 4

Comment

The clinical picture of lumbar disc prolapse is initial back pain which later radiates to the leg; with nerve root compression there is skin parasthesia, muscle cramps and tenderness progressing to sensory loss and motor weakness. If urinary and/or anal sphincter tone is compromised ('cauda equina' syndrome) emergency surgical decompression is required.

Answer 3

(a) Loosening of the prosthesis
Dislocation of the prosthesis
Osteomyelitis of the surgical site 3

(b) Clinical examination:
overlying tissue induration and joint tenderness
sinus formation

Marks

limb shortening
restriction of movements

Plain radiology of the joint:
prosthetic dislocation
prosthetic loosening
prosthetic migration
bone resorption
ostemomyelitis 3

(c) Poor surgical technique: bone infection, misplacement, nerve and muscle damage
Flawed prosthetic material: loosening or fracture of prosthesis, rapid wear of components due to foreign body reaction
Bone demineralization: fracture at site of implant 4

Comment
Hip replacement surgery is now commonplace, with long patient waiting lists for the procedure; complications of surgery are becoming increasingly familiar to carers outside as well as within the orthopaedic speciality. Joint replacement is designed to relieve pain and provide a degree of mobility with a functional lifespan of 15–20 years; the complications become increasingly prevalent with the passage of time. The development of precision implants which do not require cement may improve long-term results.

Answer 4

(a) (i) Hallux valgus deformity with inflammatory arthritis of the first metatarso-phalangeal joint 2

(ii) Symptoms are due to pressure/friction on the medial aspect of the first metatarsal head, producing joint deviation, exostosis formation and arthritis 2

(b) Habitual wearing of narrow, unyielding, raised-heel shoes that produce progressive lateral deviation of the big toe 2

(c) Surgery for hallux valgus is designed to correct the deformity and to preserve the function of the big toe; this is achieved by

Marks

excision of the medial bony prominence, division of the contracted abductor muscle of the first web space, tightening of the stretched medial collateral ligament and re-alignment of the first metatarsal shaft by wedge osteotomy 4

Comment

Conservative measures to correct hallux valgus deformity by changing to shoes with wide fronts and low heels are generally unsatisfactory, due to poor patient compliance. In severe deformities there is over- or under-riding of the second toe by the first. The former may produce a painful dorsal callosity on the second toe, or it may be displaced to impinge with and cross the third toe.

Answer 5

(a) Cervical spondylosis: this is a degenerative disease producing osteophytes which project into the intervertebral foramen; sudden neck movements or strain may precipitate symptoms, produced by the narrowed foramen on the issuing nerve root 3

(b) The lesion usually affects the nerve roots at C5/C6 or C6/C7 intervertebral joints to produce the following clinical picture: pain and/or sensory loss over shoulder tip, upper arm and dorsum of forearm (fingers are affected in C7 root involvement); weakness of trapezius, biceps and forearm extensors, and diminished biceps, triceps and supinator reflexes 3

(c) Mild symptoms may be controlled by a semi-rigid collar, analgesics and muscle relaxants; progressive neurological signs may require an anterior decompression laminectomy, with stabilization of the cervical spine with bone grafts 4

Comment

Cervical spondylosis may be asymptomatic and only come to light following neck trauma. Measures to relieve muscle spasm by partially immobilizing the cervical spine are usually sufficient until the inflammation produced by the injury subsides.

Progressive root compression affecting the use of that limb is an indication for surgical decompression. **Marks**

Answer 6

(a) Muscle spasm resulting in restricted range of movements, namely of abduction and internal rotation. A soft tissue swelling may be present 3

(b) (i) Perthes' disease (osteochondritis of the femoral epiphysis): collapse/fragmentation of ossification centre resulting in flattening of femoral head

(ii) Slipped upper femoral epiphysis: displacement of femoral epiphysis

(iii) Tuberculosis of the hip. Loss of bone density adjacent to joint with narrowing of joint space; later bone destruction, with abscess formation 4

(c) In Perthes' disease and slipped epiphysis, avascular necrosis leads to progressive deformity and osteoarthritis in early adult life

In tuberculosis, complete destruction of the joint, with abscess and later sinus formation; systemic spread may lead to a fatal outcome 3

Comment

The pathogenesis of Perthes' disease and slipped upper femoral epiphysis is ischaemia of the femoral head. Both occur between the ages of 5–15 years, when the femoral head depends on the lateral epiphyseal vessels for its blood supply. Tuberculosis of the hip joint is usually secondary to primary disease in the lung or the bowel and is accompanied by constitutional symptoms. A CXR and a positive Mantoux test are required to support the diagnosis.

Answer 7 **Marks**

(a) Injury is dependent on the extent of rotation and is progressive as follows: Tear of anterior part of lateral ligament leads to fractures of lateral malleolus and then medial malleolus (bimalleolar fracture). Tear of the medial ligament leads to fracture of posterior articular surface of tibia which may extend to a trimalleolar fracture dislocation (Pott's fracture) 4

(b) Proximal fibular fracture with diastasis of the inferior tibio-fibular joint and disruption of the interosseous tibio-fibular ligament 2

(c) Principle: restoration of normal ankle mortice
Unstable ankle fractures may be treated with

- external reduction and immobilization in above-knee plaster cast; weightbearing is avoided for 4–6 weeks
- internal fixation: (this prevents late displacement) and early mobilization 4

Comment
One of the most common diagnostic errors in ankle injuries is to miss a proximal fibular fracture; X-rays must include the knee and ankle joints. Failure of effective treatment of ankle diastasis leads to permanent ankle instability.

Answer 8

(a) (i) Rheumatoid arthritis 1

(ii) Stage 1 – synovitis: thickening of capsule, villous formation of synovium and a cell rich effusion into the joint and tendon sheaths
Stage 2 – destruction: articular cartilage, and tendon sheaths are eroded
Stage 3 – deformity: the combination of articular destruction, capsular stretching and tendon rupture leads to progressive instability and deformity of the joint 3

(b)	Normocytic, hypochromic anaemia Rise in ESR, C reactive protein and oncoproteins Rheumatoid factor present in 80% and antinuclear factor in 30% of patients	**Marks** 3
(c)	Stop synovitis, prevent deformity, reconstruct the joint and rehabilitate the patient, using a multidisciplinary approach	3

Comment

There is no cure for rheumatoid arthritis. Joint pain and swelling due to the synovitis is reduced by bed rest and non-steroidal anti-inflammatory agents. Systemic corticosteroids give effective relief of symptoms but have serious side effects. Intra-synovial injections of corticosteroids and cytotoxic drugs reduce joint inflammation, as do systemically administered gold, penicillamine, hydroxychloroquine and methotrexate (immunosuppression). Joint splinting, physiotherapy and postural training may prevent progressive deformity. Deformity associated with loss of function and pain is treated by joint reconstruction or joint replacement.

Answer 9

(a)	Decreased joint space due to thinning of cartilage Subarticular sclerosis Subchondral cyst formation Osteophyte formation	3
(b)	Analgesics and warmth Non-steroidal anti-inflammatory agents Preservation of movement by non-weightbearing exercises Adjustment of activities to reduce stress on the hip	3
(c) (i)	Progressive increase in pain Severe restriction of activities Marked deformity Progressive loss of movement, in particular abduction Radiological signs of joint destruction	3
(ii)	Total hip replacement	1

Marks

Comment
Primary osteoarthritis is common in the fifth and sixth decades of life and has no apparent underlying cause. The articular cartilage becomes soft and fibrillated, and the underlying bone shows cyst formation and sclerosis. Synovial hypertrophy and capsular fibrosis cause joint stiffness. Re-alignment osteotomy may arrest or slow further cartilage destruction, whilst arthrodesis of the hip produces freedom from pain and stability, at the expense of mobility. Total replacement arthroplasty replacing the acetabulum as well as the head of the femur is the operation of choice. 1

Answer 10

(a) Closed reduction under general anaesthetic with longitudinal traction on forearm, gradually flexing the elbow
Correct lateral displacement during traction
Monitor radial pulse throughout
Apply a back slab to flexed elbow, and a collar and cuff
Admit overnight to monitor limb circulation
Immobilize for three weeks 4

(b) Ischaemia of forearm and hand due to arterial injury, arterial spasm or swelling of flexor compartment
Treatment: remove all dressings
Reduce fracture immediately
Do not overflex a badly swollen arm
If the radial pulse does not return, surgical decompression of the forearm and/or exploration of the brachial artery at the vicinity of the fracture 3

(c) Injury to brachial artery/vein
Injury to nerves
Epiphyseal damage
Stiffness and delayed functional recovery
Volkmann's ischaemic contracture 3

Comment
The importance of this fracture is the associated neuro-vascular injury. Monitoring the radial pulse during and immediately after reduction is of cardinal importance in avoiding ischaemic injury.

Pulse, hand sensation and finger movements must be monitored, preferably overnight, to detect possible nerve or vessel compression. If closed reduction is not possible without compromising the brachial artery, open reduction or Dunlop traction (longitudinal traction via a pin in the olecranon) may be used. **Marks**

Answer 11

(a) The condition must be looked for during routine examination of the newborn
Abduct both hips with knees and hips flexed to a right angle – the 'click' of reduction of a subluxated/dislocated hip is diagnostic
Subluxated hips are reduced and maintained in abduction with double nappies
Dislocated hips are reduced and held in an abduction splint (frog plaster spica) 5

(b) Joint laxity due to unfavourable intrauterine posture, or genetic or placental hormonal factors
Dysplasia of the hip with deficient acetabulum and/or femoral head 2

(c) Treatment of established condition is difficult due to adaptive changes
Reduction of hip by closed or open method and maintained for at least six weeks
Any residual deformity is corrected by osteotomy. Acetabular dysplasia may require surgical correction at a later stage 3

Comment

Subluxated hips are not uncommon at birth (5–10 per 1000). Most reduce spontaneously soon after birth. Failure to diagnose and correct the dislocation before the child starts walking is negligent, as a good result is then difficult to achieve; osteoarthritis is a likely late complication.

Answer 12

Marks

(a) (i) Acute osteomyelitis of the radius/ulna — 1

(ii) Aspirate from area of maximal inflammation and send fluid for Gram staining and culture to identify the causative organism and its sensitivity
Raised WBC, ESR and anti-staphylococcal antibody titres — 3

(b) Cellulitis of the forearm
Acute suppurative arthritis of elbow
Sickle cell crisis
Gaucher's disease (pseudo-osteitis) — 3

(c) Analgesia and rehydration
Splint the forearm
Antibiotic therapy; initially broad spectrum, later sensitivity specific
Surgical drainage if abscess has formed — 3

Comment

Plain X-rays are of limited value during the first few days, as there is little or no radiological abnormality of the bone. By the end of the second week, periosteal new bone formation and metaphyseal mottling may be present – the classic radiological signs of pyogenic osteomyelitis: treatment should never be delayed while waiting for these signs to appear. Cellulitis of the forearm may present an identical clinical picture and, in tropical climates, pyomyositis (inflammation of skeletal muscle) is caused by the same organisms. Accompanying septicaemia and fever may cause severe dehydration, and intravenous fluids may be required.

Answer 13

(a) (i) Childhood rickets — 1

(ii) Radiology: thickening and widening of epiphysis, cupping of the metaphysis, bowing of diaphysi — 2

Marks

(iii) Biochemistry: reduced serum Ca^{++} and PO_4^{---}
($Ca \times PO_4 < 2.4$ diagnostic)
Raised serum alkaline phosphatase 2

(b) (i) Underexposure to sunlight
Vitamin D deficiency from poor diet (or post-gastrectomy in adults) or malabsorption due to coeliac or pancreatic disease or small bowel surgery
Chronic liver or kidney disease 3

(ii) Dietary vitamin D supplementation with α-calcidol (vitamin D analogue) or calciferol (vitamin D_2) up to 40,000 units daily 2

Comment

In children bowing of the tibia if marked may require the wearing of callipers to prevent further deformity and to restore normal alignment until new bone formation occurs. In adults the deficiency manifests as osteomalacia. The bones become deformed with an accompanying muscle weakness; correction of the deformities is by osteotomy.

Answer 14

(a) (i) Paget's disease of the spine (osteitis deformans) 1

(ii) Areas of osteoclastic activity with bone reabsorption, giving a radiological flame-shaped lesion along the shaft of bone
Adjacent areas of osteoblastic activity, with new bone formation, leading to radiological sclerosis and coarse trabeculation 2
Fibrovascular tissue is laid down in areas of bone excavation 4

(b) Spinal stenosis with nerve root compression
Pathological fracture
Osteoarthritis
Bone sarcoma 2

Marks

(c) Non-steroidal anti-inflammatory agents for bone and joint pain. Suppression of bone turnover by calcitonin and diphosphorates – effective when the disease is in active phase
Calcitonin decreases osteoclastic activity
Diphosphorates reduce bone growth by binding to hydroxyapatite crystals — 3

Comment

Most people with Paget's disease of the bone are asymptomatic, and the disease comes to light during X-ray investigation for an unrelated condition. Surgery is reserved for complications of pathological fractures (internal fixation with straightening of the bone) and for nerve entrapment due to severe spinal stenosis (surgical decompression). Osteogenic sarcoma, if detected early, may be resectable. A high output cardiac failure and hypercalcaemia may also be associated with the disease.

Answer 15

(a) (i) Tuberculosis of the dorsal spine (Pott's disease of the spine) — 1

(ii) Destruction of adjacent vertebral bodies by caseation leads to collapse, producing spinal angulation. The paravertebral abscess tracks down deep to the psoas fascia and points in the groin — 2

(b) Mantoux/Heaf skin test – positive
Raised ESR
CXR – evidence of primary lung lesion
X-ray of entire spine – to detect distant occult lesions and to assess the degree of angulation and the number of vertebrae and disc spaces involved at the kyphosis
CT or MRI scan for evidence of impending cord compression
Needle aspiration of the groin abscess for histological and bacteriological confirmation — 3

(c) (i) Eradicate the disease with anti-tuberculous chemotherapy
Correct deformity and prevent spinal complications by — 4

	drainage of paravertebral abscess and evacuation of infected/necrotic material Correction of angulation with strut (rib) grafts and spinal fusion Physiotherapy of the affected joints. High protein diet	**Marks** 3
(ii)	Pott's paraplegia	1

Comment

There is usually a long history of poor health and backache. Occasionally the patient may present with paraesthesia and weakness of the legs. Spinal tuberculosis should be distinguished from other causes of vertebral destruction, i.e. pyogenic infections and malignant disease. Tumour metastases may cause vertebral body collapse but, in contrast to tuberculous spondylitis, the disc space is usually preserved.

Answer 16

(a)	(i)	Acute osteomyelitis of radius/ulna Acute pyomyositis of flexor/extensor muscles	2
	(ii)	The forearm is held still across the chest with the elbow flexed Elbow and wrist movements are present, though the range of movements is restricted due to muscle spasm or bone pain	2
(b)	(i)	*Staphylococcus aureus* *Streptococcus pyogenes* *Haemophilus influenzae* Pneumococcus Salmonella	2
	(ii)	Acute osteomyelitis and pyomyositis in the early phase respond well to antibiotic therapy Sensitivity-specific agents are used once the organisms are isolated Generally, however, IV cloxacillin 200 mg/kg daily in	

Marks

divided doses – followed once the infection is under control by oral flucloxacillin 100 mg daily
In penicillin allergies, a cephalosporin or fusidic acid and erythromycin may be substituted
Malnutrition must be treated with urgent dietary measures
No surgical measures are required in the early acute phase of either illness
Abscess formation requires drainage, and bone necrosis may occur in chronic osteomyelitis with involucrum formation, when surgical debridement is required 4

Comment

The aetiology of myositis and osteomyelitis is associated with a multitude of predisposing factors. Systemic bacterial infections, e.g. staphylococcal bacteraemia, may lead to seeding of the blood-borne organism in damaged or ischaemic muscle or bone. The presence of avitaminosis and malnutrition may lead to digestive enzyme deficiencies and chronic bowel infections with an overgrowth of intestinal organisms, namely *Staphylococcus aureus*, being linked with muscle and bone infections in these children.

CHAPTER 4: NEUROSURGERY

Answer 1 **Marks**

(a) Right-sided cerebral abscess
Chronic infections from the para-nasal sinuses produce a thrombophlebitis that may extend into the cranium through the cribiform plate and infect the subdural space, resulting in an abscess 3

(b) CT or MRI scan which may be contrast-enhanced 2

(c) Aspiration of the abscess under stereotactic control and i.v. antibiotic therapy guided by the culture and sensitivity result of the aspirated pus; if the abscess is large or multi-loculated, drainage through a craniotomy may provide access for breaking down loculi and irrigation of the subdural space 5

Comment
Intracranial abscesses may arise extradurally, subdurally or within the brain. Scalp infection or an open skull fracture may directly infect the extradural space, whilst a thrombophlebitis of the cerebral veins from a middle ear or a sinus infection may infect the subdural space. This is more likely in the immunocompromised patient.

Answer 2

(a) Astrocytoma
Ependymoma
Oligodendroglioma
Medulloblastoma 2

(b) Burr hole biopsy under ultrasound guidance 2

(c) Surgical excision: complete, in circumscribed/accessible tumours; partial, in extensive/inaccessible tumours
Adjuvant therapy: radiotherapy/chemotherapy to treat residual disease
Aim: to achieve a cure, alleviate symptoms and restore neurological function 6

Comment **Marks**

An anatomic diagnosis of a brain tumour is usually made on clinical and imaging evidence; this determines surgical access and potential complications from involvement of adjacent structures. Histological verification is usually by open biopsy and is not always feasible due to the hazards of this procedure. Surgical excision may be limited due to possible neurological sequelae, but adjuvant radiotherapy or chemotherapy may give good palliation, depending on the tumour type and its malignant potential.

Answer 3

(a) Electroencephalogram
Magnetic resonance imaging (MRI) of the brain
Videotelemetry of cerebral activity 3

(b) Failure of an adequate trial of anticonvulsant drug therapy increased to the highest tolerable dosage
Surgical access with localization of the seizure focus
Evidence that surgery would improve overall quality of life
Absence of psychiatric illness 4

(c) Patients (and carers) should be informed of the following:

- post-operative psychological morbidity – usually transient; rarely, personality changes may persist
- seizures may not be completely abolished following surgery; however, there is a reduction in their frequency and duration
- co-exisiting personality disorders would not be improved but post-ictal psychosis may respond favourably 3

Comment

The clinical examination of patients with epilepsy is frequently normal. Focal lesions producing seizures are often the result of ischaemic episodes, haemorrhage or tumours.

Marks

Electroencephalography and videotelemetric monitoring of brain activity localizes the source of abnormal neuronal activity and, in conjunction with cerebral imaging, assists in planning surgical treatment. The principle of seizure surgery is excision of an identifiable focal cerebral lesion; intra-operative electrocorticography and cortical stimulation under local anaesthesia identifies the limits of surgical excision, particularly when involving the dominant cerebral hemisphere.

Answer 4

(a) (i) Infantile hydrocephalus 1

(ii) Tense anterior fontanelle
'Cracked pot' sound on percussion
Transillumination of cranial cavity
'Setting sun' appearance of the eyes
Thin scalp with dilated veins
Abnormally large skull compared with normal growth charts 3

(iii) CT or MRI head scan 1

(b) (i) Stenosis of aqueduct of Sylvius causes a sustained rise in intracranial pressure

(ii) Spina bifida
Meningomyelocele 2

(c) Cerebrospinal fluid shunt with a one-way valve between the lateral ventricle and right atrium or peritoneum 3

Comment

Hydrocephalus may be diagnosed prenatally by ultrasonography. Treatment of infantile hydrocephalus is by shunting, except in the rare chronic (arrested) hydrocephalus, where the cerebrospinal fluid pressure has returned to normal. These children require careful neurological follow-up to detect any deterioration. Following shunting, ventricular size can be monitored by ultrasonography through the open anterior fontanelle. The overall prognosis is poor, with one-third dying and one-third achieving a semblance of normality by the age of 10 years. **Marks**

Answer 5

(a) (i) Intracranial space-occupying lesion 1

(ii) Raised intracranial pressure due to tumour mass with or without obstruction of cerebrospinal fluid circulation
Fits may be due to mass effect or pressure on motor pathways 3

(b) (i) Cranial CT or MRI scan
Cerebral angiography 2

(ii) Herniation of the brain stem into the foramen magnum 1

(c) Benign tumours:
Meningioma
Acoustic neuroma
Haemangioblastoma
Epidermoid and dermoid cysts
Colloid cyst of the third ventricle

Malignant tumours:
Neuroepithelial tumour
Germ cell tumour
Lymphomas and leukaemias
Metastatic tumours 3

Comment

Epilepsy is the most frequent initial symptom of a glioma or meningioma. Headaches that are present on waking, on changing posture, coughing, straining or of unusual intensity, and occurring in those not previously prone to headaches merit CT scanning. Changes in personality, cognitive function and memory are also features suggestive of brain tumour.

Answer 6 **Marks**

(a) (i) Subarachnoid haemorrhage due to ruptured cerebral aneurysm or arterio-venous malformation 2

(ii) Increasing drowsiness leading to stupor and coma simultaneously mild focal neurological deficit may progress to moderate and then severe hemiparesis leading to decerebrate rigidity 3

(b) (i) CT or MRI head scan 1

(ii) Xanthochromia and sterile CSF 1

(c) Medical measures:
Bed rest, sedation and adequate analgesia
Treat hypertension when present
Maintain fluid and electrolyte balance

Surgery:
Control bleeding by clipping the aneurysm or feeding vessels to arterio-venous malformation 3

Comment
A sudden bleed into the subarachnoid space is soon followed by cerebral oedema and a raised intra-cranial pressure. Lumbar puncture in these circumstances may cause coning; if, however, fulminant meningitis cannot be ruled out, it may be carried out once the intra-cranial pressure stabilizes. Nimodipine, a calcium channel blocker, reduces the incidence of infarction and ischaemic deficits when administered soon after the haemorrhage.

Answer 7

(a) (i) Right hemiparesis/hemiplegia
Dysphasia
Right-sided sensory disturbance 2

(ii) Hypertension; polycythaemia; diabetes mellitus;

Marks

alcoholism; smoking; hyperlipidaemia
Atrial fibrillation or valvular heart disease 2

(b) Cranial CT or MRI scan to evaluate the extent of cerebral infarction and oedema, and presence of intra-cranial haemorrhage
Maintain airway
Anticoagulation with IV heparin 40,000 units/24 hours if cause is embolic/thrombotic
Lower raised intra-cranial pressure: positive pressure ventilation with 5% PCO_2
Reduce cerebral oedema: Mannitol infusion and/or corticosteroid therapy
Maintain fluid, electrolyte and acid-base balance 6

Comment
Investigations should be directed towards categorizing the vascular event as a guide to prognosis. Surgical measures for improving cerebral perfusion or for cerebral decompression do not generally improve prognosis. Surgery may have a role in preventing subsequent stroke in those who survive the initial event.

Answer 8

(a) A history of a prodromal period with malaise, fever and listlessness
Clinical features of an underlying source of infection
Focal neurological signs (including epileptic fits)
Change in level of consciousness, i.e. drowsiness or irritability 3

(b) (i) Streptococcus
Staphylococcus aureus
Proteus
Bacteroides fragilis
Escherichia coli
Haemophilus influenzae 2

Marks

(ii) Bronchitis/pneumonia
Otitis media
Sinus infection
Gastroenteritis 2

(c) Correct fluid and electrolyte balance
Sedation
Initially broad spectrum antimicrobial therapy then specific agent(s) once pus culture and sensitivity are available
Surgical aspiration or excision 3

Comment

A brain abscess is a mass lesion producing focal neurological signs and must be distinguished from meningitis. Lumbar puncture is contraindicated due to the danger of tentorial herniation. Antibiotic therapy: the initial choice of antibiotic before culture results are available will depend on the probable cause of the abscess and the Gram stain.

Aspiration of an abscess may be performed by use of CT-guided stereotaxis. Aspiration may need to be repeated with CT follow-up. Surgical excision is indicated:

- For persistent re-accumulation despite repeated aspirations
- If the abscess is not accessible for aspiration
- In the presence of a fibrous capsule surrounding the abscess preventing collapse on aspiration.

Answer 9

(a) Cervical cord lesion causing compression: extradural abscess; metastatic tumours; intradural tumours, e.g. meningioma, Schwannoma; intramedullary tumours, e.g. gliomas

Spinal lesions causing compression: cervical spondylolisthesis/spondylitis; intervertebral disc prolapse; infections of vertebral body (e.g. Pott's disease) 3

		Marks
(b)	Muscle wasting and lower motor neurone weakness, with sensory disturbance of nerve roots C5 to T1	3
(c)	(i) Plain cervical spine X-rays Myelography CT scan (with intrathecal contrast) or MRI	2
	(ii) Mild symptoms due to degenerative lesions of the spine respond well to analgesics, rest, physiotherapy and wearing of a collar Surgical decompression of the cervical cord is required occasionally as an emergency for progressive neurological signs Radiotherapy with corticosteroids is indicated for malignant cord compression	2

Comment

A feature of spinal cord compression is local and radicular pain which predates sensory and motor disturbances. Urinary sphincter disturbances may also be present. The tingling, or 'electric shock' sensation on flexion/extension of the neck (Lhemitte's sign) is diagnostic. Metastatic tumour deposits are from the lung, breast, kidney and prostate. Tumours of the reticulo-endothelial system also metastasise to the spine. Urgent surgery is required for progressive neurological signs to avoid permanent disability. Local palliative radiotherapy in malignant disease relieves pain and may produce a partial remission of weakness. It may be as effective in metastatic disease as surgical decompression.

CHAPTER 5: EYES, ENT AND SKIN

Answer 1 **Marks**

(a)	Cancrum oris (noma)	2
(b)	Protein–calorie malnutrition Chronic anaemia (? hookwork infestation) Measles Poor oral hygiene during the period of tooth eruption	3
(c)	Parenteral broad-spectrum antibiotic therapy Naso-gastric feeding of high protein–calorie diet Antiseptic mouthwash and wound irrigation Closure of defect following healing with a cutaneous pedicled flap transfer	5

Comment

This is a necrotizing stomatitis or a severe form of ulcerative gingivitis arising from the gums and spreading to the mandible and to the cheek, resulting in a gaping hole in the side of the face; the child is at risk of developing overwhelming sepsis. The infection must, therefore, be treated urgently with i.v. penicillin and metronidazole and frequent wound irrigation. The accompanying malnutrition must be corrected; a blood transfusion may be required to correct severe anaemia. Surgery is deferred until healing and involves excision of the contracture (which produces trismus) and a pedicled skin flap closure of the defect.

Answer 2

(a)	(i) Acute recurrent tonsillitis	2
	(ii) Adenoidal hypertrophy	2
(b)	Palpable cervical lymph node (tonsillar node) largyngoscopy; tonsils swollen, inflamed and indurated; pus may be expressed from the tonsillar crypts	3
(c)	Tonsillectomy and adenoidectomy under antibiotic cover	3

Comment **Marks**

Adenoidal hypertrophy is a frequent accompaniment of tonsillar hypertrophy from recurrent bacterial infection, and is implicated in obstructive sleep apnoea syndrome and sudden infant death syndrome. The indications for tonsillectomy are recurrent attacks of tonsillitis (>3 episodes/year), peritonsillar abscess (quinsy) and chronic tonsillitis, particularly if associated with respiratory, cardiac, renal or rheumatic illness. Indications for adenoidectomy are recurrent middle ear infection, post-nasal obstruction or discharge, or recurrent sinusitis 4

Answer 3

(a) (i) Burkitt's lymphoma 2

(ii) Plain radiology of the facial bones
Intra-oral biopsy 2

(b) (i) Affects pre-adolescent children confined to the equatorial belt of 4° latitude, which includes the tropica rain forest

(ii) The Epstein–Barr virus

(iii) Chronic malnutrition 3

(c) Oral cyclophosphamide alone or in combination 3

Comment

This is a childhood tumour confined to a geographical belt which implicates environmental factors in its causation. It was first studied in children in equatorial Africa, but is also found in New Guinea and Central America. The tumour arises from the jaw, close to the alveolar margin, with radiological signs of its disruption. The response to cyclophosphamide is usually rapid with the tumour virtually 'melting away' within a few weeks.

Answer 4 **Marks**

(a) Squamous carcinoma (Marjolin's ulcer)
An ulcerating lesion, minimally tender, with an indurated base and everted edges; surrounded by thin or hypertrophic scar tissue; popliteal or groin lymphadenopathy; may be palpable 4

(b) Incisional biopsy from edge of ulcer 2

(c) Excision of the ulcer with a 2 cm clear margin extending down to the fascia and split skin or pedicled flap grafting
Block dissection of the groin nodes if found to contain tumour following sentinel node biopsy 4

Comment

When a squamous carcinoma develops in a cutaneous scar, it is usually as a result of poor healing or chronic irritation. It differs from other skin cancers in that it is relatively painless and grows slowly over a prolonged period; distant metastases are delayed due to the paucity of blood supply and lymphatic drainage in scar tissue. During surgical excision it is advisable to include as much of the surrounding scar tissue as possible.

Answer 5

(a) Occlusion of central retinal artery or vein
Ischaemic optic neuropathy
Retinal detachment
Vitreous haemorrhage
Temporal arteritis
Hysterical blindness
Macular lesions 4

(b) Atherosclerosis
Hypertension
Diabetes mellitus 3

(c) Any lesion involving the optic chiasma, including ischaemic infarction
Hysterical blindness 3

Marks

Comment

The fundus in central retinal artery occlusion is creamy white due to an infarcted retina, except over the macula, which is visible as 'the cherry red spot'. In ischaemic optic neuropathy (due to temporal arteritis), a pale and swollen optic disc is present; in retinal detachment the opaque retina obscures the normal choroidal red glow, and instead there is a grey, rippling reflex.

Answer 6

(a) Conjunctivitis
Episcleritis and scleritis
Keratitis
Uveitis — 2

(b) Look for a foreign body in the conjunctiva
Pupillary reflexes to light
Slit lamp examination of iris and lens
Fundoscopic examination of the retina
Fluorescein stain for corneal abrasions/ulcer — 4

(c) Retinoblastoma:
Enucleation with chemo and/or radiotherapy — 4

Comment

Red eye in the adult: three major causes are iritis, keratitis and acute angle closure (acute glaucoma). Signs on slit lamp examination are ciliary injection and white deposits on the corneal surface in iritis; a broken corneal epithelium in keratitis; and a hazy cornea with a shallow anterior chamber and a dilated pupil in acute glaucoma.

Answer 7

(a) (i) Acute orbital cellulitis — 1

(ii) Conjunctival and nasopharyngeal swabs for culture and sensitivity
Aerobic and anaerobic blood cultures
AP and lateral X-rays of paranasal sinuses and orbit — 2

			Marks
(b)	(i)	Broad spectrum IV antibiotic therapy changing if required to sensitivity-specific IV rehydration Pain relief and sedation as required	2
	(ii)	Place on a pulse and temperature chart Test visual acuity and pupillary reaction twice daily and examine the optic disc daily Serial ultrasound or CT scan to detect early signs of subperiosteal abscess formation	2
(c)	(i)	Surgical drainage and/or excision of the ethmoidal sinus, with drainage of frontal and sphenoidal sinuses	2
	(ii)	Cavernous sinus thrombosis, which may lead to a brain abscess	1

Comment

Acute orbital cellulitis is the most common cause of exophthalmos in children and usually spreads from an infected ethmoid sinus. Preseptal cellulitis, which is a common complication of acute sinusitis, may spread to the orbit, as orbital septa are not well developed in children. Following recovery on antibiotic therapy, the underlying paranasal sinusitis must be treated to prevent recurrences. Orbital surgical exploration is required if the infection cannot be controlled by antibiotics, with the danger of the infection spreading to the globe (panophthalmitis).

Answer 8

(a)	(i)	Blow-out fracture of the orbital floor	1
	(ii)	A hard object larger than 5 cm in diameter striking the orbit causes a sudden increase in intraorbital pressure, which produces orbital floor fracture	2
(b)	(i)	Infraorbital nerve injury causes anaesthesia involving the lower eyelid, cheek, side of nose, upper lip and teeth. Diplopia, when present, is typically vertical in both up-and-down gaze and is caused by tethering of extra-ocular	

Marks

muscles to the fracture line. Enophthalmos may be present initially or may appear later as the periorbital oedema subsides and the eyeball sinks into the fractured floor 3

(ii) Plain orbital X-rays (Waters' view)
CT scan of orbit (axial and coronal sections) 1

(c) Small cracks in the orbital floor without diplopia require no treatment. Fractures of less than 50% of the floor, with improving diplopia, require no treatment unless enophthalmos is more than 2 mm. Fractures of over 50% of the floor, with persistent diplopia, should be repaired within two weeks of injury 3

Comment
Despite the invariable presence of conjunctival ecchymosis and chemosis, orbital injuries rarely cause ocular damage. Surgical treatment of orbital floor fractures entails freeing the entrapped tissue and covering the defect with a plastic plate. Orbital margins offer little protection to small missiles, such as squash balls and shuttlecocks that may impact directly onto the eyeball and cause serious ocular injury.

Answer 9

(a) Chronic laryngitis due to vocal abuse, tobacco use or myxoedema
Laryngeal polyps, nodules, granulomas and papillomas 2

(b) Indirect laryngoscopy by use of a laryngeal mirror with or without pharyngeal anaesthetic spray
Fibreoptic laryngoscopy via nostril with topical anaesthetic spray
Direct laryngoscopy under general anaesthetic (e.g. in children) 4

(c) Radiotherapy for most early lesions – with a cure rate of 90%
Laser beam surgical excision of early lesions is also curative

Marks

For extensive cord carcinomas, a partial or total laryngectomy may be performed in conjunction with a neck dissection for nodal involvement
Total laryngectomy requires a tracheostomy and oesophageal voice training — 4

Comment

Laryngeal nodules, a specific and localized form of chronic laryngitis, are found in professional voice users (singer's nodules) and in children (screamer's nodules). Juvenile papillomas must be excluded in hoarseness in children; they are due to the human papilloma virus.

Carcinomas may present above (supra-glottic) or below (infra-glottic) the vocal cords. They have a worse prognosis than glottic tumours, as hoarseness is a late symptom and diagnosis being delayed until the cord is involved; the greater vascularity and lymphatic drainage above and below the cord predisposes to earlier metastases.

Answer 10

(a) (i) Conductive deafness caused by secretory otitis media is due to Eustachian tube dysfunction — 2

(ii) Predisposition:
Acute otitis media
Adenoidal inflammation
Post-nasal space neoplasm
Barotrauma — 2

(b) There is reduced mobility of the eardrum, with hyperaemia
The middle ear effusion may alter in composition and appear golden-brown or blue
Occasionally bubbles may be seen through the drum
A retracted drum with prominent malleus and occasional vesicles — 2

Marks

(c) Myringotomy: aspiration of fluid under a general anaesthetic if troublesome symptoms persist for over three months
Insertion of a grommet (a tiny flanged Teflon tube) into the drum is frequently required to avoid recurrence of middle ear fluid
An anterior or inferior radial myringotomy incision is used to insert the grommet — 4

Comment

Secretory otitis media may settle spontaneously. Nasal vasoconstrictor drops with an oral decongestant may assist recovery when there is an associated upper respiratory tract infection.

A marked and persistent hearing loss interfering with schooling necessitates surgery. This may involve the insertion of a grommet to drain and ventilate the middle ear. The grommet usually extrudes spontaneously 6–18 months after insertion. If normal Eustachian tube function has not returned and secretory otitis media recurs, the grommet is replaced.

Answer 11

(a) (i) The lesion: the edge, base, floor and surrounding skin
Regional lymph nodes — 1

(ii) Malignant melanoma — 1

(iii) Depth of invasion is measured from the top of the granular layer of the epidermis to the deepest melanoma cell in the dermis
Tumour thickness < 0.76 mm has a favourable prognosis — 2

(b) Wide local excision down to deep fascia
If histologically malignant:
Sentinel node biopsy
Radiotherapy with/without nodal clearance and/or chemotherapy based on histological staging or distant spread — 3

Marks

(c) Protection from sun by clothing and wide-brimmed hats Apply sun screen lotions containing skin protection factors and limit time of exposure 3

Comment

Malignant change in a pre-existing naevus is difficult to assess as there is uncertainty whether melanomas always arise from pigmented moles. However, a change in size, itchiness or bleeding should arouse suspicion. Delayed or missed diagnosis may result in dissemination, though it is unclear if this occurs during the radial or vertical growth phases. Diagnosis is by histological examination of the whole lesion, and incisional biopsy is, therefore, ill-advised.

Answer 12

(a) Basal cell carcinoma
Malignant melanoma
Squamous cell carcinoma 3

(b) Excision for histological confirmation with adequate surrounding clearance. Plastic surgery may be required to close the defect. Cryosurgery or curettage and cautery are suited for small lesions. Radiotherapy for basal cell carcinoma is an option when surgery would be poorly tolerated 4

(c) (i) Ultraviolet light on certain skin types produces dysplasia of epidermal cell layers leading to actinic keratosis; this may progress to invasive tumours 2

(ii) Wearing protective clothing and headgear; limit exposure to direct sunlight and apply sun screen lotions during exposure 1

Comment

The choice of treatment for facial lesions is based on the size of the tumour and on the physical state of the patient, as well as on cosmetic considerations. In general, surgery is preferred for those lesions that can be totally excised and the skin closed with minimal cosmetic disfigurement.

Marks

Interestingly, most melanomas occur on skin that is only intermittently exposed to the sun; individuals with higher continuous exposure have lower rates than those exposed intermittently, and curiously, the use of sunscreens may increase rather than decrease the melanoma risk. Most dysplastic lesions do not progress to skin malignancy; some may regress with time.

CHAPTER 6: ENDOCRINOLOGY, BREAST AND CHEST

Answer 1 **Marks**

(a) (i) Goitre
Parathyroid adenoma
Thyroglossal cyst
Cervical lymph adenopathy
Branchial cyst
Dermoid and epidermal cysts 2

(ii) Thyroid and parathyroid glands:
move with swelling
Thyroglossal cyst: lies over hyoid bone
Branchial cyst: lies near angle of mandible
Lymph nodes: usually lateral to the mid-line and
may be multiple 2

(b) Neck and thoracic inlet views
Ultrasound, radioisotope scan
Thyroid function tests, serum Ca^{++}
FNAC 2

(c) Thyroid cancer, or when malignancy cannot be excluded
Dyspnoea due to tracheal deviation/compression
Toxicity non-responsiveness to antithyroid agents
Retrosternal extension
Cosmetic considerations 4

Comment

A swelling located over the thyroid cartilage is almost invariably a goitre and requires functional assessment. Branchial and thyroglossal cysts require excision as they are liable to beome infected and symptomatic. Enlarged cervical lymph nodes are caused by a host of local and systemic factors, and node biopsy may be required to assess in diagnosis or treatment. Thyroid cancers are treated surgically by total or near-total thyroidectomy, except for some anaplastic tumours and lymphomas. The latter respond well to chemotherapy, whereas in the former, the response to any form of treatment is poor.

Answer 2 **Marks**

(a) (i) Thyrotoxicosis 1

(ii) Proptosis; lid lag; lid retraction
Fine tremor; rapid sleeping pulse
Thyroid bruit, functional systolic murmur 3

(b) TSH, T3, T4
^{131}I thyroid scan 3

(c) Inpatient monitoring of pulse, BP and respiration
Anti-thyroid drugs (e.g. carbimazole)
Anti-arrhythmic agents (e.g. propranolol)
Night sedation (e.g. nitrazepam)
Subtotal thyroidectomy when the patient is euthyroid
Lugol's iodine is administered for a few days pre-operatively 3

Comment
Subtotal thyroidectomy is the treatment of choice for thyrotoxicosis; anti-thyroid agents may lead to recurrence of symptoms following cessation of treatment; radio-iodine therapy leads to hypothyroidism over a period of time and is contraindicated in young adults. In the presence of eye signs the condition is referred to as Graves' disease. Eye signs rarely respond to medical measures or subtotal thyroidectomy. Orbital decompression or tarsorraphy may be required for cosmetic purposes and occasionally for conjuntivitis and chemosis.

Answer 3

(a) Texture and firmness of goitre
Retrosternal extension
Pain on palpation
Presence of palpable neck nodes suggests papillary, medullary or anaplastic tumours
Palpable bony lesions suggest follicular or anaplastic carcinoma 3

		Marks
(b)	Thyroid malignancy invading the larynx or the recurrent laryngeal nerve causing vocal cord palsy Indirect laryngoscopy	2
(c)	(i) Ultrasound scan of the thyroid with guided FNAC X-ray of neck and thoracic inlet ^{131}I uptake thyroid scan	3
	(ii) Poor or no uptake of isotope ^{131}I in a discrete area suggests absence of functional thyroid tissue. This may represent a cystic lesion or a solid lesion, e.g. a follicular adenoma or a carcinoma	2

Comment

Papillary carcinomas account for 60% of all thyroid malignancies and have a good prognosis, despite nodal recurrence. Lymphatic spread also occurs in medullary (C-cell) and anaplastic carcinomas but blood-borne spread is common, and the prognosis poor. Calcitonin is produced by medullary tumours and is used as a tumour marker to detect recurrence following total thyroidectomy.

Answer 4

(a)	Ca^{++} and phosphate are lost from bone due to loss of renal tubular reabsorption, leading to osteoporosis	3
(b)	Fall in serum Ca^{++} due to urinary loss stimulates PTH secretion and, if sustained, leads to parathyroid hyperplasia	3
(c)	Removal of all parathyroid glands and place patient on long-term α-calciferol (vitamin D analogue) therapy	4

Comment

In primary hyperparathyroidism the increased PTH production is due to primary hyperplasia, an adenoma or, rarely, a carcinoma of the parathyroid. Treatment consists of removal of all four glands, when hyperplasic, with possible re-implantation of a portion of one gland in a surgically accessible site. When removing a functional adenoma or a carcinoma the other glands are usually hypoplastic and do not require removal. **Marks**

Secondary hyperparathyroidism is due to a sustained low serum Ca^{++} level from any cause. Re-establishing normal serum Ca^{++} should lead to resolution of the hyperplastic state, though this is uncommon in chronic renal failure.

In tertiary hyperparathyroidism PTH production becomes independent of serum Ca^{++} levels, and the glands become autonomous, leading to hypercalcaemic states. Total parathyroidectomy and vitamin D analogue administration brings about homeostasis.

Answer 5

(a) (i) Phaeochromocytoma 1

(ii) Serum and urinary noradrenaline and/or adrenaline levels would be elevated 2

(b) (i) The catecholamines secreted by the tumour produce cardiovascular instability, i.e. hypertension and cardiac arrhythmias 2

(ii) α-blockade by phenoxybenzamine (20–80 mg daily in divided doses) lowers the BP
β-blockade by propranolol (120–140 mg daily in divided doses) converts cardiac irregularities to sinus rhythm 3

(iii) Adrenalectomy 2

Comment
Phaeochromocytomas are neuro-ectodermal tumours of the sympathetic chain, 90% of which arise in the adrenal gland, and the remainder elsewhere along the chain. Most tumours release both adrenaline and noradrenaline but large tumours produce only noradrenaline. Scanning with ^{131}I or ^{132}I metaiodobenzylguanidine (MMIBG) produces specific uptake in sites of sympathetic activity and is used for diagnostic confirmation. Adrenal surgery must be supported by α and β blockade (the former preceding the latter),

along with whole-blood transfusion as required to re-expand the contracted intravascular volume. **Marks**

Answer 6

(a) (i) Cushing's disease or syndrome 1

(ii) Dexamethasone suppression test 1

(b) (i) Pituitary gland or adrenal gland 1

(ii) High resolution CT scan with IV contrast or MRI scan 1

(iii) Pituitary gland:
gigantism or acromegaly
hyperprolactinaemic syndrome
thyrotoxicosis
Adrenal gland:
phaeochromocytoma
Conn's syndrome
Addison's disease 3

(c) Medical treatment with anti-secretory drugs
Surgical removal of pituitary tumour by trans-sphenoidal hypophysectomy
Radiotherapy if surgical excision is incomplete 3

Comment

Cushing's disease is due to an adrenocorticotropin (ACTH)-secreting pituitary tumour, resulting in bilateral adrenocortical hyperplasia and secretion of adrenal corticosteroids. Cushing's syndrome is due to an adrenal tumour or to a cortisol-secreting ectopic source, such as a bronchial carcinoma. The diagnosis of Cushing's disease is based on a failure of the pituitary source of ACTH to be suppressed by dexamethasone. Corticotrophin-releasing hormone given to those with a pituitary source of ACTH results in a normal or exaggerated corticotrophin or cortisol response, but adrenal tumours or ectopic sources of ACTH do not respond.

Answer 7 **Marks**

(a) (i) Express nipple discharge
Thickening/eczema of nipple; peau d'orange
Palpable lesion underlying the nipple areolar complex 2

(ii) Supraclavicular nodes
Axillary nodes
Liver enlargement
Contralateral breast 2

(iii) Intraduct papilloma
Ductal carcinoma *in situ* (DCIS)
Duct ectasia 3

(b) Cytology on nipple discharge
Mammography and/or U/S scan
FNAC of a palpable lesion
Wire-guided excision biopsy 3

Comment

Duct papilloma, common between the ages of 35–50 years, usually presents with a blood-stained nipple discharge as the only symptom. On examination a lump may be felt beneath the areola. Removal of the papilloma and the involved duct (microdochectomy) or ducts (major duct excision) is curative. However, a ductal carcinoma may have an identical clinical presentation and would necessitate a mastectomy following biopsy confirmation.

Answer 8

(a) (i) Size, consistency and mobility of lump
Attachment to overlying skin or chest wall 2

(ii) Axillary nodes
Supraclavicular nodes
Internal mammary chain
Inferior epigastric chain 2

		Marks
(b)	Ultrasound Mammogram FNAC; core needle biopsy	2
(c)	Removal of the entire breast or part, with axillary nodal sampling/clearance Radiotherapy Chemotherapy Hormonal manipulation	4

Comment

FNA cytology, ultrasonographic and mammographic findings are graded from benign to obviously malignant. When all three parameters show high grades for malignancy, breast ablation may be safely undertaken. Otherwise, histological confirmation on biopsy must be awaited. The 'frozen section biopsy, query proceed to mastectomy' scenario is less often seen today, as a delay of a few days between tumour biopsy and mastectomy does not adversely alter the prognosis. This allows for better emotional and psychological preparation of the patient. Counselling for breast reconstruction is required if the patient requests reconstruction at the time of the mastectomy.

Answer 9

(a)	(i)	Infiltrating ductal (scirrhous) carcinoma	1
	(ii)	Palpate right axilla and supraclavicular fossa Examine contralateral breast and abdomen CXR and bone scan Liver scan and pelvic ultrasound examination	3
(b)	(i)	Yes	1
	(ii)	Wide local excision, with tamoxifen	2
	(iii)	The lesion may persist unchanged for a considerable period of time before metastasising. It is possible she may die in the meantime of an unrelated cause	3

Marks

Comment

Scirrhous tumours in the elderly are usually slow growing and slow to metastasise. Surgical treatment, therefore, should be confined to local removal. If surgery is declined, a course of radiotherapy, with tamoxifen, may shrink the tumour and improve the prognosis. There is little place for adjunct chemotherapy. Approximately half to one-third of these tumours are oestrogen receptor positive and respond favourably to tamoxifen alone.

Answer 10

(a) Mammography (or obtain screening mammograms)
Ultrasound scan of breast
Image-guided FNAC — 3

(b) LFT; CXR
Ultrasound and/or isotope liver scan
Radionucleide bone scan
Bone marrow aspiration biopsy
Brain scan (only if indicated) — 3

(c) Mastectomy or breast-conserving surgery for peripherally sited tumours with axillary clearance
Radiotherapy to the breast following wide local excision and to the axilla (instead of axillary surgery)
Adjuvant chemotherapy for distant spread is based on tumour grade and nodal status — 4

Comment

Palpable and impalpable breast lesions may be graded by mammography and ultrasonography as well as by cytology to determine malignancy. If these findings are equivocal, stereotactic guided wire localization enables impalpable lesions to be located and removed for histology. Definitive cancer surgery should not be performed on the basis of any one positive parameter, i.e. clinical, cytological or imaging (positive cytology must be supported by ultrasonography and mammography or core needle biopsy). Breast-conserving operations remove small, unifocal cancers (less than 4 cm in size). Axillary node dissection is mainly for the staging of the disease for adjuvant therapy.

Answer 11 **Marks**

(a) (i) Congenital diaphragmatic hernia 1

(ii) Mediastinal shift to the right
Presence of bowel and/or gastric gas shadows in left pleural cavity
Collapse/compression of left lung 3

(b) Acute respiratory distress due to gastric dilatation leading to collapse and consolidation of the affected lung
Volvulus of herniated stomach
Acute bowel obstruction may lead to perforation of herniated bowel loop 3

(c) Surgical reduction of abdominal contents from the pleural cavity and excision of the herniated sac
Repair of defect in left diaphragm
Re-expansion of left lung
Ventilatory support in the post-operative period 3

Comment

The usual sites of congenital diaphragmatic herniae are the foramen of Bochdalek (pleuro-peritoneal hernia), oesophageal hiatus, foramen of Morgagni (anteriorly) and the dome. The condition must be distinguished from acute respiratory distress syndrome, oesophageal atresia and hypertrophic pyloric stenosis. Occasionally the child may present with impending or actual obstruction of the herniated bowel loop. Radiological features are, therefore, important in establishing the diagnosis.

Answer 12

(a) General anaesthesia: left lateral position with right arm supported on an arm rest
Aseptic skin preparation
Insertion of fibre-optic scope into pleural space through a laterally placed stab incision in the second to the fifth intercostal space

	Marks
Structures visualized: lung surface, adhesions and fluid in pleural space Pleural biopsies and fluid aspiration	3
(b) Pre-op workup, including lung function studies Single lung anaesthesia Thoracotomy: decortication with evacuation of inflammatory tissue and pus Tissue samples sent for histology, and microbiological culture, including TB	4
(c) Complication of chronic lung infections, e.g. lung abscess Organisms: TB, *Staphylococcus aureus* Iatrogenic introduction of infection into pleural space (during diagnostic needle aspiration)	3

Comment

The thoracoscopy would have been preceded by CXR and CT or MRI scans to localize the primary lesion in the lung. A primary tumour of the lung or pleura may give rise to these symptoms but a pyogenic or tubercular lung lesion is more common. In immunocompromised patients, chronic lung infections with atypical organisms frequently lead to pulmonary complications, such as abscess formation and empyema.

Answer 13

(a) Papillary carcinoma of thyroid Bronchial carcinoma Breast carcinoma Gastric carcinoma Pancreatic carcinoma	2
(b) Bronchial small cell carcinoma CXR (postero-anterior including lateral views) Sputum for cytology Bronchoscopy with brush and tissue biopsies for cytology and histology, respectively Whole body CT scan for metastases	4

Marks

(c) Removal of primary tumour (lobectomy or pneumonectomy) and regional lymph nodes
Adjuvant chemotherapy — 4

Comment
Small cell carcinomas account for 15% and squamous and adenocarcinomas for 70% of all lung cancers. Mediastinoscopy for nodal visualization and biopsy indicates the extent of mediastinal nodal involvement by tumour. When contralateral nodes are involved surgery is ill-advised. Only 20% of patients with lung cancer are considered suitable for surgery. The majority receive palliation with chemotherapy.

Answer 14

(a) (i) Ischaemic heart disease — 1

(ii) ECG, Echocardiogram — 1

(iii) Ischaemic changes in pre-cordial leads
Myocardial and valvular functional defects — 2

(b) Coronary angiography defines the site(s), extent and degree of stenosis and treatment involves balloon angioplasty and/or insertion of coronary stents to revascularize diseased vessels — 3

(c) Coronary artery bypass grafting (CABG) of diseased vessels using the internal mammary or the gastro-epiploic artery or the long saphenous vein. The operation is performed by use of extracorporeal circulation, with systemic anticoagulation — 3

Comment
Balloon angioplasty and CABG have been shown to significantly reduce myocardial infarcts in patients with critical cardiac ischaemia. Bypass grafting is indicated when the angiogram shows extensive narrowing of two or more coronary vessels not amenable to angioplasty.

CHAPTER 7: UPPER ALIMENTARY TRACT

Answer 1 **Marks**

(a) Troisier's sign: nodal metastases at the root of the neck, usually from a gastric carcinoma
FNAC or biopsy of the node may reveal an adenocarcinoma originating from the upper gastrointestinal tract 2

(b) Gastroscopy and mucosal biopsy
Double-contrast barium meal
CT or MRI scan 3

(c) Macroscopically recognized types are:
Type 1 – cauliflower-like lesion
Type 2 – ulcer-cancer
Type 3 – colloid carcinoma
Type 4 – scirrhous carcinoma (linitis plastica)
Type 5 – carcinoma in a previously benign gastric ulcer

Definitive treatment:
Localized lesions (types 1, 2 and 5) – partial or subtotal gastrectomy
Diffuse lesions (types 3 and 4) – total gastrectomy

Palliative treatment:
Unresectable lesions – surgical bypass or endoscopic intubation to facilitate gastric emptying
chemotherapy 5

Comment

Gastric cancers usually present insidiously or with a diversity of symptoms; there appears to be a considerable time lapse between the appearance of the cancer and its clinical manifestations. Pancreatic tumours also have a similar presentation. Laparoscopy assesses feasibility of resection. Radical surgery for the early lesion, which includes removal of the regional lymph nodes, offers the best hope of a cure. The presentation of an epigastric mass lesion with/without jaundice indicates an advanced lesion with impending gastric outlet or biliary obstruction. Bypass surgery with chemotherapy offers the best palliation.

Answer 2 **Marks**

(a) (i) Pleomorphic adenoma of parotid gland 1

(ii) Size and location
Per oral examination of fauces for involvement of deep part of gland
Involvement of branches of the facial nerve 3

(b) Contraindicated due to seeding of tumour along the needle track to skin 2

(c) (i) A conservative superficial parotidectomy (conservative total parotidectomy with preservation of the facial nerve branches if the deep part of the gland is involved) 3

(ii) Facial nerve trunk and its five branches must be preserved 1

Comment
Pleomorphic adenomas are locally invasive and 'shelling out' the tumour invariably leads to recurrence; re-exploration may compromise the facial nerve and its branches. Dissection of the facial nerve branches during removal of the deep portion of the gland leads to transient facial palsy in the post-operative perod and is due to neuropraxia from bruising or tissue swelling.

Answer 3

(a) (i) Ludwig's angina (acute cellulitis of the submandibular and cervical regions)
Inflammation and swelling of tissue planes superficial and deep to the investing layer of the deep cervical fascia, involving the submandibular region 2

(ii) Streptococcal species
Vincent's organisms
Gram-negative anaerobes 2

Marks

(b) (i) The inflammatory oedema extends deep to the investing layer of deep cervical fascia at and above the level of the hyoid bone, involving the glottis and displacing the tongue upwards and out through the mouth, leading to the imminent danger of asphyxiation — 2

(ii) Rehydration and analgesia
IV amoxycillin or a cephalosporin with metronidazole gives broad spectrum therapy and usually leads to rapid resolution

If resolution is delayed, surgical decompression and drainage of the submandibular space under local infiltration anaesthesia is required — 4

Comment

Ludwig's angina is an infection of a closed fascial space and, if untreated, the inflammatory exudate may track along the stylohyoid muscle to the submucosa of the glottis, when the patient is in danger of asphyxiation from glottic oedema.

Surgical decompression is through a curved incision beneath the mandible, displacing the submandibular gland and dividing the mylohyoid muscles, thereby opening up the fascial space.

Answer 4

(a) Dysphagia for solids and/or liquids
Pain on swallowing
Retrosternal pain/discomfort
Vomiting old food
Aspirating saliva leading to recurrent chest infections
Site of obstruction as felt by patient — 2

(b) (i) Bulbar (and pseudobulbar) palsy
Extra-oesophageal compression due to mediastinal tumours
Iron deficiency anaemia
Pharyngeal pouch

Marks

Oesophageal causes:
scleroderma
inflammatory stricture
malignant stricture
achalasia — 3

(ii) Barium swallow: outlines the lesion and defines the anatomical site
OGD: Visualization and biopsy of lesion — 2

(c) Aetiology: Hiatus hernia produces reflux oesophagitis and stricture
Malignant stricture: smoking and alcohol or Barrett's oesophagus produces squamous metaplasia and may lead to anaplasia — 3

Comment

The oesophagus is inaccessible to clinical examination; consequently, a working diagnosis of oesophageal cancer must be based on the presenting symptoms and confirmed by endoscopy or imaging. Occasionally a patient may present with respiratory symptoms due to aspiration or tumour extension into the trachea or bronchus. Surgery is aimed at removing the tumour and restoring continuity by bringing the stomach up into the chest or by interposing a loop of large bowel. Radiotherapy is a viable treatment option, as squamous carcinomas are radiosensitive.

Adenocarcinomas of the gastric fundus may extend into the oesophagus, producing dysphagia. Surgery entails an oesophago-proximal gastrectomy and resytoring continuity, using either the distal gastric remnant or a jejunal Roux loop.

Answer 5

(a) (i) Peptic ulcer disease — 1

(ii) Stressful lifestyle
Helicobacter pylori infection
Alcohol and smoking
Irregular meals — 2

		Marks
(b)	OGD Sedation (2–5 mg IV midazolam) Mouth guard and anaesthetic throat spray Visualization through endoscope or on video screen Endoscopic biopsy via biopsy channel	2
(c)	(i) Adopt healthy life style measures Stop oral intake of anti-inflammatory agents Eradication of *H. pylori* by broad-spectrum antibiotics (amoxycillin and clarithromycin or metronidazole) with H_2-receptor blockade (cimetidine, ranitidine), or proton pump inhibition (omeprazole or lansoprazole) Surgery (anti-acid procedure) for failed medical therapy and for complications	3
	(ii) Complications of peptic ulceration: bleeding, perforation, stenosis causing gastric outlet obstruction Chronic pre-pyloric ulceration may predispose to gastric carcinoma	2

Comment

The importance of stress, alcohol and tobacco in the aetiology of this disease requires the implementation of 'life style measures' aimed at reducing these factors and promoting health.

Since the advent of effective medical measures in ulcer healing, surgery for peptic ulcer disease is reserved for the complications of bleeding, perforation, stenosis and possible malignancy.

An anti-ulcer procedure involves denerving the stomach (vagotomy) and draining the denervated stomach (by a pyloroplasty or a gastro-enterostomy) or removing the acid secreting portion of the stomach (antrectomy or distal gastrectomy).

Answer 6

(a)	(i) Hypertrophic pyloric stenosis	2
	(ii) Achalasia of the cardia	

	Marks
Duodenal atresia Annular pancreas	2
(iii) The hypertrophied pylorus ('pyloric tumour')	1
(b) Hypertrophy of the circular smooth muscle fibres of the pylorus producing a functional gastric outlet obstruction	2
(c) Medical measures: rehydration; smooth muscle relaxants (e.g. hyocine) prior to feeds Surgery: division of all hypertrophied muscle fibres without breaching the mucosa	3

Comment

The palpation of an enlarged pylorus following a feed, with the infant preferably asleep, is diagnostic of hypertrophic stenosis and imaging is unnecessary. Medical measures are not generally successful.

Answer 7

(a) (i) Oesophageal atresia with/without tracheo-oesophageal fistula	1
(ii) Gastrograffin swallow	1

(b) (i)

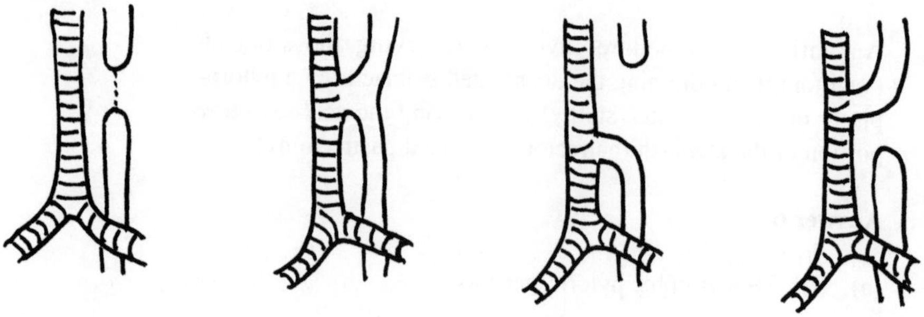

		Marks
	(ii) Passage of nasal feeding tube into stomach to confirm oesophageal patency by aspirating stomach contents	2
(c)	Transthoracic excision of oesophageal atresia and associated tracheo-oesophageal fistula, with restoration of oesophageal continuity and repair of tracheal defect	2

Comment
Oesophageal atresia must be diagnosed at birth to prevent the aspiration pneumonitis that rapidly ensues. The simple procedure of passing a nasal feeding catheter and the insertion of a rectal thermometer at birth brings to light developmental abnormalities at each end of the alimentary tract.

Answer 8

(a)	(i)	Hiatus hernia	1
	(ii)	Herniation of portion of stomach into left pleural cavity leading to a sliding or rolling hernia resulting in oesophageal ulceration and bleeding, and later oesophageal stricture in the former. Squamous metaplasia may occur in the portion of stomach that slides into the chest, giving rise to Barrett's oesophagus, a premalignant condition	3
	(iii)	Barium swallow or OGD	1
(b)	(i)	Erect and semi-recumbent posture at work and sleep Anti-reflux medication (alginate preparations, antacids) Reduce gastric acid production with H_2-receptor blockade Weight reduction	2
	(ii)	An anti-reflux operation, such as the Nissen fundoplication or the Leigh Collis gastroplasty performed through the abdomen, or the Belsey repair performed through the chest	3

Comment **Marks**

Treatment of hiatus hernia is aimed at relief of symptoms. A dramatic improvement occurs following weight reduction in those who are overweight. Many operations have been devised as none have been entirely satisfactory. The Nissen fundoplication is probably the procedure most often used and may now be performed laparoscopically.

Answer 9

(a) Test for the presence of urease (Cloe test) for evidence of *Helicobacter pylori*

Haematoxylin and eosin stain for evidence of type II gastritis and/or the presence of *H. pylori*
Culture isolation 3

(b) (i) *Helicobacter pylori* 1

(ii) Treatment regimes involve gastric acid suppression and antibiotic therapy; these include clarithromycin 500 mg b.i.d. and either omeprazole 20 mg b.i.d. or lansoprazole 500 mg b.i.d. and either metronidazole 400 mg b.i.d. or tinidazole 500 mg b.i.d. 3

(c) *Helicobacter pylori* is found in Type II gastritis. It raises the local pH by ammonia production and may thereby cause mucosal damage, leading to ulceration. The persistence of infection leads to chronicity and gastric ulcers may predispose to malignancy 2

Comment

Helicobacter pylori infection has been implicated in the aetiology of peptic ulcer disease. H_2-receptor or calcium channel blockers reduce gastric acid production, but to achieve permanent ulcer healing, eradication of the underlying *Helicobacter pylori* infection and the chronic gastritis it produces is required.

Answer 10	**Marks**
(a) Immediate control of bleeding by Sangstaken–Blakemore tube placement, or Endoscopic sclerotherapy and IV vasopressin If these measures fail, consider oesophageal transection or emergency porta-systemic shunt	4
(b) Chronic liver damage (e.g. hepatitis B infection or alcohol abuse) predisposes to cirrhosis, which in turn leads to portal hypertension and variceal bleeding	3
(c) Three- to six-monthly follow-up oesophagoscopy and prophylactic sclerotherapy or banding of recurrent varices. Long-term follow-up is mandatory	3

Comment

Treatment of gastro-oesophageal varices is palliative unless the underlying portal hypertension is curable. Elective surgical shunts (spleno-renal, mesocaval and porta-caval) require satisfactory liver function (Child's groups A and B) to be effective. In selected cases orthopic liver transplantation has been successful.

Answer 11

(a) (i) Peritonitis due to peptic ulcer perforation	2
(ii) Free gas on erect abdominal X-ray, i.e. under right diaphragm and between bowel loops Inflammatory thickening of the pro-peritoneal fat layer in the abdominal wall	2
(b) IV analgesia and antibiotics IV fluids; nasogastric aspiration Consent for emergency laparotomy Closure of perforation and peritoneal toilet with definitive anti-ulcer surgery in selected patients	4
(c) Stop or change anti-inflammatory agent to one less ulcergenic Commence long-term anti-ulcer medication	2

Comment **Marks**

Emergency surgery is mandatory in a perforated viscus due to the lethal complications of peritonitis. In a young and otherwise fit patient with a peptic perforation, recurrent ulceration may be prevented by an anti-ulcer operation during the emergency surgery. Very occasionally a 'pin hole' perforation with limited peritoneal contamination may be non-surgically managed in the expectation that the perforation would seal itself; close monitoring is then essential to assess response.

Answer 12

(a) Primary haemorrhage: during surgery, from uncontrolled bleeding points
Reactionary haemorrhage following return to normal BP
Secondary haemorrhage occurs a few days later, due to infection 3

(b) Quarter-hourly blood pressure, pulse and respiratory rate and central venous pressure monitoring
Examination of abdominal wound and abdominal girth measurement
Resuscitation if required
Blood volume replacement
Emergency surgical re-exploration and haemostasis 4

(c) Pneumococcal infection due to fall in cell-mediated immunity
Prophylaxis: pneumovaccine
Antibiotic (penicillin V) cover for future invasive procedures 3

Comment

Post-operative bleeding from uncontrolled bleeding points into body cavities, such as the chest and abdomen, may go unnoticed until the patient lapses into oligaemic shock. Suitably placed drains assist in its early detection, and close monitoring of vital signs enables timely resuscitation and surgical control.

To preserve immunological functions of the spleen, a small portion of the spleen may be re-implanted during splenectomy for splenic trauma. **Marks**

Answer 13

(a) An ulcer with slough on an indurated base and everted edges
Pain
Salivation
Ankyloglossia
Dysphagia
Inability to articulate clearly
Alteration in the voice
Fetor oris
Lump in the neck due to cervical nodal spread 3

(b) Leucoplakia
Smoking
Spirits
Spices
Sepsis
Friction (from sharp edge of tooth)
Syphilis
Candidiasis 3

(c) *In situ* and small (<1 cm) tumours are excised with a 1 cm clear margin. Lesions <2 cm are treated by interstitial irradiation by use of caesium needles or iridium wire.
For lesions >2 cm external beam irradiation is used.
Tumours with cervical nodal metastases are treated with a combination of radiotherapy and block dissection of the neck nodes. 4

Comment
Leucoplakia is regarded as a pre-cancerous condition. When causative irritants are identified and avoided, early lesions disappear. Surgical excision of cancerous lesions on the tongue is limited due to the resulting functional disability. Except for the very small lesions, all tongue cancers are treated with radiotherapy. The place of chemotherapy is undecided.

CHAPTER 8: LIVER, GALL BLADDER AND PANCREAS

Answer 1 **Marks**

(a) Infective:
- malaria
- schistosomiasis
- hydatid disease
- kala-azar

Blood dyscrasias:
- chronic leukaemia
- polycythaemia rubra vera
- sickle-cell disease
- thalassaemia
- hereditary spherocytosis

Circulatory:
- portal hypertension

Autoimmune disease:
- Felty's syndrome
- Still's syndrome

Neoplastic:
- Hodgkin's and non-Hodgkin's lymphomas 3

(b) Hypersplenism is splenic enlargement with the sequestration and/or destruction of peripheral blood cells in the splenic circulation; this results in anaemia, leukopenia and/or thrombocytopenia 3

(c) A grossly enlarged spleen is at an increased risk of rupture, 1 either spontaneously or following mild trauma; the medical indications are:

- hypersplenism
- hereditary spherocytosis
- idiopathic thrombocytopenic purpura
- autoimmune haemolytic anaemias
- Felty's syndrome
- tropical splenomegaly syndrome

Marks

hydatid disease
schistosomiasis
staging of Hodgkin's disease
primary splenic tumours
pyruvate kinase deficiency 4

Comment

A grossly enlarged spleen is invariably associated with hypersplenism and is also prone to rupture from blunt trauma. Elective splenectomy is indicated for the correction of specific haematological abnormalities, in the treatment of some blood cancers and in the staging of Hodgkin's disease.

Answer 2

(a) (i) Calculus cholecystitis 1

(ii) Murphy's sign
Palpable gall bladder
Paraesthesia over the right upper quadrant and back 2

(iii) Ultrasound scan of the gall bladder and biliary tree 1

(b) Increasing concentrations of cholesterol, bile pigments and lecithin in the bile, with a reduction in the bile acid pool leads to cholesterol, pigment and calcium salt supersaturation. In the absence of glycoprotein crystallization inhibitors and impaired gall bladder motility and/or infection, these compounds crystallize to form stones 3

(c) Remove inflamed gall bladder by open or laparoscopic cholecystectomy. During the procedure image for stones in the biliary tree by per-operative cholangiogram and explore the bile duct if indicated 3

Comment 2

The classical symptoms of cholecystitis that follow a fatty meal are due to cholecystokinin secreted by the presence of fat in the duodenum stimulating a diseased gall bladder to contract, usually against a stone. Non-functioning gall bladders, despite containing stones, may remain silent for this reason. There is, therefore, no indication for treating asymptomatic gall stones. **Marks**

Answer 3

(a) (i) Ascending cholangitis 1

(ii) Migration of gall stones from gall bladder into bile duct $\rightarrow$ obstruction $\rightarrow$ biliary stasis $\rightarrow$ ascending infection 2

(iii) Hb and WBC detect anaemia and sepsis
LFT indicate extent of liver damage by obstruction to bile flow and sepsis
Serum amylase, if elevated, suggests pancreatic duct obstruction, with pancreatitis
Blood cultures: aerobic and anaerobic may isolate offending organism(s) 3

(b) Ultrasound and imino-diacepic acid excretion scans of the liver and biliary tree 1

(c) Rehydration with IV fluids
Analgesia
Correct anaemia
Treat infection with IV antibiotics
Drain biliary tree by percutaneous transhepatic catheter, ERCP and endoscopic sphincterotomy, or surgical drainage of bile duct, with cholecystectomy 3

Comment
Cholangiohepatitis in Western societies is caused by ascending infection due to migrating gall stones obstructing the common bile duct. It is important to distinguish this from viral hepatitis, which is largely a self-limiting illness. As progressive liver damage occurs, the biliary tree must be decompressed as an emergency, by means of a transhepatic catheter. Planned surgical or endoscopic drainage should follow.

Marks

Answer 4

(a) (i) Accidental injury or ligation of the common hepatic or bile duct — 1

(ii) Percutaneous transhepatic cholangiogram (PTC) — 1

(iii) CXR, coagulation screen
Vitamin K prophylaxis
Blood group and cross-match — 2

(b) Biliary leak causing peritonitis due to partial/complete division of the bile duct — 2

(c) Good exposure and visualization of the surgical field
Identification of anatomy of Callot's triangle
Per-operative cholangiogram
Immediate T-tube drainage following accidental injury to bile duct — 4

Comment
Damage to the hepatic or bile ducts during cholecystectomy is an avoidable catastrophe. Technical inexpertise, along with the occasionally encountered anomalies of the hepatic artery and ducts, account for the majority of these misadventures. During laparoscopic cholecystectomy the surgeon should, on encountering technical difficulty, convert to an open operation. Per-operative cholangiogram assists in outlining the anatomy in a difficult dissection.

Answer 5

(a) (i) Gall stone ileus — 1

(ii) Chronic calculus cholecystitis leading to erosion of the gall stone into the duodenum and its passage down the small bowel, with obstruction usually in the distal ileum — 1

		Marks
(iii)	Distended loops of small bowel Possible radio-opaque calculus in terminal ileum Air in the biliary tree	2
(b)	Nasogastric aspiration Fluid and electrolyte replacement Adequate analgesia Emergency laparotomy and relief of obstruction with cholecystecomy	3
(c)	Ultrasound scan of gall bladder and biliary tree to confirm calculus disease and assess calibre of bile duct ERCP and sphincterotomy if duct stones are present	3

Comment

Gall stone ileus is an uncommon complication of cholelithiasis and, as a history of biliary disease may not be obvious (a proportion of gall stones being silent), air in the biliary tree on abdominal X-ray usually clarifies the diagnosis. When removing the gall bladder, it may be found to be firmly adherent to the duodenum, and a duodenal fistula may require closure.

Answer 6

(a)	(i) Acute pancreatitis	1
	(ii) Biliary calculi Alcohol abuse	2

(b) Resuscitate:

oxygen by face mask or nasal catheter
IV fluids
pain relief
nasogastric aspiration
IV broad-spectrum antibiotics

Monitor:

Lung function and tissue oxygenation: respiratory rate and arterial blood gas estimation
Circulation: BP, pulse rate and CVP measurement

	Marks
Liver and kidney function: U&E, LFT and urine output Pancreatic function: blood glucose and serum and urinary calcium estimations	4
(c) Hypovolaemic shock Respiratory failure Renal failure Secondary infection Pseudocyst formation Hypocalcaemia	3

Comment

The course of acute pancreatitis is unpredictable, irrespective of the underlying cause. In a small minority of patients the disease is rapidly progressive, and early identification of this group enables close monitoring and support of cardio-respiratory and renal functions in an intensive care setting. Surgical intervention is restricted to complications of pancreatic haemorrhage or necrosis in fulminant disease, or of abscess or pseudo-cyst formation in subacute disease.

Answer 7

(a) Periampullary carcinoma or bile duct carcinoma Pancreatic, biliary and liver imaging by ultrasound and CT ERCP Cytology on pancreatic juice and bile obtained at ERCP Percutaneous image guided core needle biopsy	3
(b) (i) Supportive and hospice care Palliation by endoscopic or transhepatic stenting of malignant stricture Surgical palliation by biliary by-pass operation Curative surgery: Pancreatoduodenectomy (Whipple's operation)	3
(ii) Poor anaesthetic or surgical risk Advanced primary tumour Local and/or regional spread of tumour	2

		Marks
(c)	Haemorrhage Wound infection Wound dehiscence Delayed wound healing Renal failure	2

Comment

Most ampullary and biliary tumours are beyond curative measures on presentation and are treated palliatively. Pain is controlled by opiates when required. Pancreatic supplements will aid digestion and reduce weight loss. Pruritus is associated with jaundice and both are relieved by stenting or bypassing the obstruction.

Answer 8

(a)	(i)	Stress ulcer (Curling's ulcer) of the stomach or duodenum Haemobilia	2
	(ii)	Stress ulcer is treated by H_2-receptor or calcium channel blockade Ulcer bleeding uncontrolled by the above measures may be treated by submucous injection of adrenaline or laser photocoagulation Haemobilia is due to a traumatic fistula between a hepatic vessel and a branch of the biliary tree. It usually resolves, otherwise angiographic embolisation of the fistula is required	4
(b)	(i)	A pancreatic fistula	1
	(ii)	A fistulogram through the drainage tube or ERCP	1
(c)	(i)	A leak from damage to the bile duct system	1
	(ii)	An imidoacetic acid excretion scan or ERCP	1

	Marks

Comment

Complications of trauma to the bile duct or pancreas may present late and represent unrecognized injury. Traumatic pancreatic fistulae close on supportive measures alone if continuity of the pancreatic duct is preserved. Complete transection, however, rarely heals without surgical intervention. Pseudocyst formation is a late complication of pancreatic injury. It resolves either spontaneously or following ultrasound-guided aspirations, provided there is no underlying pancreatic disease.

Answer 9

			Marks
(a)	(i)	A clinical label when an underlying causative factor has not been found	1
	(ii)	Obsessive-compulsive neuroses Attention-seeking behaviour patterns Anorexia nervosa and bulimic disorders	2
(b)	(i)	Chronic relapsing pancreatitis A raised serum amylase A normal or low serum calcium AXR may show pancreatic calcification Abdominal U/S scan may show pancreatic calculi, fibrosis or oedema	3
	(ii)	Abstinence from alcohol and a low fat diet with pancreatic enzyme supplementation. When pain persists, despite patient compliance, it is usually due to fibrosis of the duct: relief may be achieved by splanchnic nerve block Long-term pain relief using narcotic analgesics may lead to habituation and drug dependency Surgical measures are restricted to complications such as chronic relapsing pancreatitis and intractable pain non-responsive to other measures	4

Comment **Marks**

Surgery is based on pancreatographic and CT findings. If the head of the pancreas is diseased, a pancreatoduodectomy is performed, with the distal segment draining into the stomach or jejunum. Involvement of the distal segment would require a distal pancreatectomy. Occasionally the duct is grossly dilated due to multiple stenoses; it is opened along its length by filleting the gland, and drained into a loop of bowel (longitudinal pancreato-jejunostomy – Peustow operation).

CHAPTER 9: SMALL AND LARGE BOWEL

Answer 1 **Marks**

(a) Adenomatosis
Inflammatory
Metaplastic
Harmatomatous 2

(b) Endoscopic assessment of whether the lesion is benign or malignant with multiple biopsies
Exclude the presence of polyps elsewhere in the colon
When the extent of the lesion makes it unsuitable for endoscopic removal, surgical resection of the involved segment of colon is advisable
Colonic surveillance follows treatment 5

(c) This patient has, in all probability, adenomatous polyps which may be familial or sporadic; familial polyposis accounts for <5% of the incidence; the remainder are sporadic
Probable associated dietary factors are high-fat, low-residue and red meat 3

Comment
Colonic polyps may be pedunculated or sessile; the risk of malignant change increases with the increasing size of the polyp. Polyps <5 cm in size may be treated endoscopically by snaring or diathermy obliteration. Large polyps, particularly when broad-based or sessil, may require surgical resection of the involved segment of bowel. Polyps, with the exception of juvenile and inflammatory polyps, are prone to recur and these patients must be kept under colonoscopic or imaging surveillance.

Answer 2

(a) Idiopathic slow transit constipation
Laxative abuse
Irritable bowel syndrome
Obstructed defecation 2

		Marks
(b)	Abdominal and rectal examination Rigid sigmoidoscopy Faecal occult bloods to screen for malignancy Whole gut transit time using a capsule containing radio-opaque markers Defecating proctography – if main symptom is difficulty in defecation	3
(c)	Wean patient off laxatives and counsel patient if there is a pattern of laxative abuse Introduce bulk into diet May require total colectomy if symptoms are unremitting	5

Comment

Chronic constipation is a common ailment of modern societies and tends to resolve with the introduction of high-fibre ingredients to the diet with bulk formers, such as Fybogel, Isogel and Lactulose. Sedentary lifestyles predispose to this condition and physical activity should be encouraged. Idiopathic slow transit constipation may not respond to dietary or medical measures, and total colectomy and ileorectal anastomosis is curative in carefully selected patients. In those with difficulty in defectation with normal transit times, a feature is pelvic floor weakness which descends on straining. Other conditions are anterior rectocele and rectal intussesception; these patients may resort to digitally assisting defecation.

Answer 3

(a)	Exacerbation of the diverticular disease Acute diverticulitis	2
(b)	Raised white cell count Raised serum C-reactive protein If there is evidence of abscess formation, surgical drainage Colonoscopy or barium enema following successful management of the acute episode	4

		Marks
(c)	Bedrest i.v. fluids and nil by mouth i.v. Gram-negative anaerobe-sensitive antibiotics (metronidazole) Colonoscopy/barium enema Surgical resection of the involved segement if there is luminal narrowing due to scarring	4

Comment

Diverticulosis is the incidental finding of diverticulae in the asymptomatic patient; diverticular disease is when patients have symptoms such as distention, flatulence and pelvic heaviness; colonic segmentation in response to food may cause pain. Diverticulitis is inflammation of the diverticulae, usually from inspissated faeces and produces persistent lower abdominal pain and peritonism when there is serosal involvement; the sigmoid colon which is involved most often is palpable and tender. The aim of management is resolution of the infection and the exclusion of a concurrent colonic malignancy.

Answer 4

(a)	(i)	Acute bowel obstruction due to intussusception	1
	(ii)	Aetiology: Lymphoid hyperplasia in bowel wall due to weaning and enteric viral infections; childhood leukaemias and bowel lymphomas	2
(b)		Abdominal examination: Distention, tympanitic, increased bowel sounds Palpable mass PR: empty ampulla, possibly a pelvic mass; ‘redcurrant jelly’ on finger stall	3
(c)	(i)	Barium or gastrograffin enema	1
	(ii)	Under a light general anaesthetic dilute barium is trickled into the rectum under a hydrostatic pressure not exceeding 30 cm of water	

	Marks
Screening identifies the position and features of the intussusception. The pressure is maintained for a period (not exceeding 30 minutes) before rescreening to assess reduction of the intussusception	3

Comment

The presence of a mobile abdominal mass with 'redcurrant jelly' stool is diagnostic of an intussusception. Diluted barium or gastrograffin reduces the intussusception by hydrostatic pressure and thereby avoids an operation. However, when the diagnosis is delayed or the presentation is late, even surgical reduction may prove difficult, due to the extensive oedema of the trapped bowel. Further, as the intussusception progresses, the blood supply is compromised, with infarction of the intussuscepted bowel loop.

Answer 5

(a)	Infective diarrhoea Inflammatory bowel disease Neoplasms, i.e. benign polyps, adenocarcinoma or lymphoma	3
(b)	Sigmoidoscopy (rigid or flexible), followed by barium enema or colonoscopy, with full bowel preparation Endoscopic mucosal biopsies	4
(c)	Ascitic tap for protein content and cytology A low protein content would exclude an inflammatory cause, and the presence of neoplastic cells would suggest a disseminated colonic cancer Liver ultrasound or radioisotope scan may reveal discrete lesions, such as a liver abscess or metastatic tumour deposits	3

Comment

Inflammatory bowel disease and bowel cancer have similar presentations. The former is incurable but compatible with a normal life expectancy, whereas the latter has a favourable prognosis if detected early and a dismal outcome when diagnosed late. Ulcerative colitis carries a small but significant risk of cancer, which increases with time. These patients must, therefore, be on colonoscopic surveillance.

Answer 6 **Marks**

(a) (i) Distended and tympanitic abdomen, minimally tender, with a possible palpable lesion
Increased bowel sounds
Empty rectum on rectal examination, with possible melaena on finger stall 2

(ii) Working diagnosis: subacute colonic obstruction due to neoplasia or adhesions 1

(b) (i) Plain abdominal X-ray (supine and erect) 1

(ii) Features: dilated small and large bowel loops
Presence of air/fluid levels, faecal impaction and possibly the shadow of a colonic lesion
A barium enema should not be performed in large bowel obstruction 2

(c) Management:
FBC, U&Es, CXR, ECG
IV rehydration
Correct anaemia
Nil by mouth
Naso-gastric aspiration if necessary
Catheterize to monitor urine output
Group and cross-match
IM analgesia
Prepare for surgical relief of bowel obstruction 4

Comment

In the middle-aged and the elderly, a malignant colonic lesion must be suspected in the absence of a history of chronic constipation, inflammatory bowel disease and post-surgical adhesions. Obstructive symptoms are delayed in proximal colonic tumours, due to the liquid nature of their contents. These patients may, therefore, present late with anaemia and weight loss due to tumour ulceration and invasion. Early diagnosis and appropriate surgical resection is curative in Duke's A and early B tumours. Some Duke's B and all C tumours require adjuvant chemotherapy. Pre-operative radiotherapy may down-stage the tumours in the treatment of rectal cancers. **Marks**

Answer 7

(a) Dilated loops of jejunum and/or ileum with air–fluid levels
Absence of gas in bowel distal to obstruction 2

(b) (i) Assessment of dehydration and electrolyte depletion: tongue moisture and skin turgor
U&E and ABG estimation for electrolyte and acid-base balance
Monitor naso-gastric aspirate (approx. 1000–2000 ml/24 hr)
Urine output (approx. 1300 ml/24 hr) and urine osmolarity
Insensible to fluid loss (approx. 700 ml/24 hr) 3

(ii) Treat deficit and daily requirements by giving isotonic (0.9%) saline alternating with 5% dextrose or with one-fifth isotonic (0.18%) saline and 4.3% dextrose solution with additional 60–100 mmol of K^+ per 24 hr (the dextrose provides 400–500 calories per 24 hr)
Twice-daily haematocrit and U&E estimation and urine output guide the daily replacement 3

(c) Drip and suck regime
Keep patient in fluid and electrolyte balance
Failure to respond to the above measures may require laparotomy and division of adhesions 2

Comment

The average adult requires 2000–3000 ml of water containing at least 100 mmol of Na^+ and 60 mmol of K^+ daily. These requirements are increased by the degree of dehydration. However, great care must be exercised not to over-transfuse for 'to overload the circulation is a grievous fault, and grievously does the patient pay for it'. If normal bowel function does not return in a few days, parenteral alimentation (intravenous feeding) must be considered to prevent the breakdown of body proteins.

Answer 8 **Marks**

(a) Hirschsprung's disease
Ano–rectal malformations (i.e. rectal atresia, rectal stenosis, imperforate anus) 2

(b) (i) Hirschsprung's disease or primary megacolon 1

(ii) Absence of ganglion cells in nerve plexus of the large bowel wall, leading to spasm of the involved segment and dilatation of the normally innervated proximal loop 3

(c) (i) Barium enema shows characteristic 'funnelling' at site of obstruction
Rectal biopsy for histological confirmation of absence of ganglion cells and/or cholinesterase staining for absence of acetylcholine 2

(ii) Exclusion of the aganglionic segment by a 'pull through' operation 2

Comment
In Hirschsprung's disease there is a complete physiological obstruction in the distal colon at or above the peritoneal reflection. Barium enema is diagnostic and demonstrates the dilated normal proximal bowel leading to a coned transitional zone and to the narrowed aganglionic zone. Those with a very short segment of aganglionic bowel may present later in childhood or, very occasionally, in adulthood.

Answer 9

(a) (i) Exomphalos (omphalocoele) 1

(ii) During intra-uterine life a portion of intestine lies outside the abdomen (between the 6th and 12th week)
Due to an error in development, the intestine fails to return to the abdomen at birth, with a resultant defect in the abdominal wall 3

		Marks
(b)	Immediate surgery aimed at reducing the contents of the sac and closing the defect in the abdomen The sac is covered with moist dressing to prevent rupture prior to surgery If closure of the abdominal defect is not possible, a silastic sheath may be sutured on to the abdominal wall until elective repair a few weeks later	3
(c)	Oesophageal atresia (with or without tracheo–oesophageal fistula) Duodenal atesia (also intestinal atresia) Imperforate anus (ano-rectal malformation)	3

Comment

Exomphalos is when a portion of the alimentary tract lies outside the abdominal cavity enclosed by the umbilical cord. It differs from gastroschisis, where the abdominal contents are exteriorized through a defect in the abdominal wall adjacent to the umbilical cord.

When these anomalies are associated with a large defect or a poorly developed abdominal wall, it is inadvisable to attempt to reduce the contents and close the defect, due to ensuing respiratory complications. It may be possible to achieve skin cover alone, or a silastic sheath may be sutured onto the opening and the contents gradually reduced by twisting the sheath over a period of time as the abdominal wall expands.

Answer 10

(a)	(i)	Ischio-rectal abscess	1
	(ii)	Anal mucosal crypt infection which persists to form a crypt abscess which then enlarges and extends into peri-anal fat; expansion in the confined ischio-rectal fossa leads to severe pain	3
(b)	(i)	Fistula *in ano*	1
	(ii)	Incision and drainage under a general anaesthetic with curettage of the abscess cavity with de-roofing	

		Marks
	The cavity is packed with ribbon gauze soaked in antiseptic	2
(iii)	Low fistulous tracts are excised or laid open. In high fistulae, i.e. those that lie above the anal sphincters, a seton of nylon or braided wire is threaded in and tied to gradually obliterate the tract. Complicated or recurrent high fistulae may require excision, with preliminary faecal diversion	3

Comment

Ischio-rectal abscess must be surgically drained on presentation. The presence of Gram-negative coliform organisms in the pus obtained suggests communication with the bowel and, rarely, biopsy of the abscess wall may reveal Crohn's disease. Medical treatment for Crohn's disease is then commenced and surgery limited to treating infective complications in the perineum. Persistent fistulae in the absence of inflammatory bowel disease are the result of recurrent peri-anal abscess formation and form tortuous tracts with multiple cutaneous openings. These may require staged surgical procedures for a cure, with a preliminary colostomy.

Answer 11

(a)	(i)	Digital rectal examination to palpate lesions in the rectum and pelvis Rigid sigmoidoscopy to visualise the rectum and distal sigmoid colon Protoscopy to visualise the ano-rectum	3
	(ii)	Carcinoma Ulcerative colitis Crohn's colitis Polyps	3
(b)	(i)	Prolapsing haemorrhoids (Other causes are ano-rectal polyps and mucosal prolapse)	1

		Marks
(ii)	Injection sclerotherapy Rubber banding Haemorrhoidectomy Cryosurgery	3

Comment

Rectal bleeding in any form should alert the clinician to the possibility of a large bowel tumour, especially in the older age group. The presence of piles (the commonest cause of bleeding PR) should not preclude a sigmoidoscopic examination, as the piles may prove to be a red herring masking a more sinister proximal lesion. In the presence of a recent alteration in bowel habit with or without weight loss, imaging of the entire colon or colonoscopy may be required to exclude an occult neoplasm. 3

Answer 12

(a) (i) General appearance: size, shape, contact bleeding, punched out, shallow or irregular
Base: indurated or soft, fixed or mobile
Edges: everted, rolled up or sloping 3

(ii) Multiple punch biopsies from the ulcer edge 2

(b) (i) Liver 1

(ii) Ultrasound or radio-isotope scan of the liver 1

(iii) Pre-operative bowel preparation
An anterior resection of the rectum and distal sigmoid colon preserving the anal canal if the tumour is above the peritoneal reflection, or a synchronised combined abdomino-perineal excision of the ano-rectum and distal sigmoid colon if the anal canal is involved 3

Comment

It is necessary to counsel the patient regarding the planned operation and the need for either a temporary or permanent colostomy, its siting and management. Sphincter-preserving operations for rectal cancer aim at restoring bowel continuity, thereby avoiding a permanent stoma of an abdomino-perineal excision. However, a 5 cm distal clearance of the tumour must be attainable to avoid tumour recurrence at the anastomosis.

CHAPTER 10: UROLOGY

Answer 1 **Marks**

(a) Ectopia vesicae 2

(b) Mucosa of the posterior bladder wall
Trigone
Ureteric orifices 3

(c) Absence of the umbilicus
Groin hernias
Separation and poor development of the pubic bones
Epispadias in the male 2

(d) Treat urinary infection
Assess and support renal function
Surgical reconstruction of the bladder, abdominal wall and the pelvic ring (preliminary urinary diversion may be required) 3

Comment
Ectopia vesicae results in the absence of the lower anterior abdominal wall and the anterior bladder wall with the posterior bladder wall fused to the margins of the abdominal wall defect. The quality of life is poor without treatment due to incontinence and recurrent urinary infection; there is also the long-term risk of bladder malignancy.

Answer 2

(a) (i) Phimosis 2

(ii) Inability to retract the foreskin, with evidence of scarring and stenosis 2

(b) Balanitis
Urethritis
Cystitis 3

(c) Circumcision 3

Comment **Marks**

True phimosis is scarring of the foreskin which does not retract without fissuring. A tight foreskin is what is usually encountered and is caused by physiological adhesions between the foreskin and the glans; these may be gradually broken down by progressive freeing of the foreskin in the bath and retracting it over the glans. Circumcision is the preferred treatment for true phimosis and prevent balanitis, recurrent urinary infection and the slight long-term risk of penile cancer.

Answer 3

(a) Vesical calculus 2

(b) Relieve retention by urethral catheter
Plain abdominal radiography
Urethro-cystoscopy or a cystogram, and a micturating urethrogram 4

(c) Removal of the calculus by lithotripsy or cystotomy 4

Comment

Bladder stones are eight times more common in males than in females and are classified into primary and secondary stones. Chronic malnutrition in children is a predisposing factor for primary stones and chronic urinary infection for secondary stones. There may be a sense of incomplete emptying or interruption of the urinary stream with strangury. Urinary infection is a common presenting symptom.

Answer 4

(a) (i) Testis, epididymis, cord structures
Tunica vaginalis, scrotal skin
Abdominal hernial contents 3

(ii) Examination:
Get above it to exclude hernia
Palpate the testis and the epididymis on its upper pole posteriorly; feel the cord structures and examine for a hydrocele 2

		Marks
(b)	(i) Teratoma, seminoma, yolk sac tumour	3
	(ii) Orchidectomy Radiotherapy to para-aortic nodes Chemotherapy	2

Comment

Scrotal swellings include vaginal hydrocele (most common), tuberculosis and tumour. Epididymo-orchitis, due to pyogenic organisms, generally have an acute presentation. When a testicular tumour is suspected, percutaneous biopsy is contra-indicated due to seeding of tumour in the needle track and spread to the groin nodes. An open biopsy with frozen section histology and proceed to orchidectomy if malignancy is confirmed.

Answer 5

(a)	Right reducible inguinal or femoral hernia Visible or tactile cough impulse above or below the inguinal ligament	3
(b)	Prostatic enlargement or urethral stricture Palpable urinary bladder Enlarged prostate on PR, or palpable stricture in penile urethra	3
(c)	Investigate urinary symptoms with flow studies IVU and/or ultrasound of urinary tract; urethro-cystoscopy Treatment: Prostatectomy or stricturoplasty and hernia repair	4

Comment

Chronic increase in intra-abdominal pressure may precipitate an abdominal hernia. Chronic obstructive airway disease, chronic constipation, ascites or an obstructive uropathy must be excluded in patients presenting with a groin hernia and the precipitating cause(s) treated before the hernia is repaired.

Answer 6 **Marks**

(a) (i) Torsion of the spermatic cord (testis) 1

(ii) Pyrexia; tender, swollen testis
Horizontal lie of testis ('dumbell sign')
Absent urethral discharge
Clear urine 3

(b) Surgical exploration with orchidopexy, if testis is non-viable perform an orchidectomy
Fix the other testis to prevent it torting 3

(c) Exploration is no longer indicated due to testicular non-viability
Antibiotics and analgesics
Observe in the ward until symptoms resolve
Testicular atrophy is the end result
The opposite testis must be fixed at an early date 3

Comment

An attempt may be made to untwist a torted testis on presentation; the immediate relief of pain indicates success. Surgical fixation should then be performed without undue delay. The opposite testis is also fixed, as the anatomical abnormality is likely to be bilateral.

Answer 7

(a) (i) Pneumaturia 1

(ii) Colo-vesical or colo-uteric fistula caused by either invasion of the urinary bladder or ureter by recurrent tumour or radiation damage 2

(b) Intravenous urography
Cytoscopy
Cystourethrogram 3

(c)	Diverticular disease Crohn's disease Bladder cancer Diabetes mellitus	**Marks** 4

Comment

Closure of the fistula is usually not possible when it is due to tumour infiltration or in the presence of post-irradiation fibrosis. Faecal diversion by fashioning a proximal defunctioning colostomy halts further contamination of the renal tract with bowel pathogens. It also facililates further irradiation of the pelvis for tumour recurrence without the risk of radiation colitis.

Answer 8

(a)	Haemorrhage from the prostatic bed with clot retention Perforation of the urinary bladder	4
(b)	Myoadenomatous hyperplasia Prostatic carcinoma	2
(c)	Bladder outflow obstruction leads to chronic retention of urine, which produces hydronephrosis and atrophy of the renal cortex, due to pressure effects and infection Prostatic cancer, when present (incidence 25% at 75 years of age), invades the capsule and may involve the pelvis with bony metastases or the rectum with fistula formation	4

Comment

Haemorrhage following prostatic surgery is usually reactionary, leading to clot retention; or secondary (usually a week after the operation) due to infection or straining. Perforation of the bladder or breaching the prostatic capsule may occur during transurethral surgery and, if not immediately recognized, leads to severe haemorrhage from the prostatic venous plexus in the latter; bladder perforation may be undetected post-operatively due to the indwelling catheter preventing extravasation of urine. Both these complications are serious and may require re-exploration under a general anaesthetic.

Answer 9 **Marks**

(a) Diabetic neuropathy
Psychosexual dysfunction
Undescended testes
Previous pelvic surgery or injury 3

(b) Sperm count
Sperm motility
Percentage of normal to abnormal cells
pH and sugar content of seminal fluid 3

(c) Tuberculous epididymo-orchitis 1

Urinalysis: microscopy and culture for tubercular bacilli
Testicular biopsy for histological and microbiological evidence of tuberculosis 3

Comment
An obvious cause of sterility is previous vasectomy and a request for surgical reversal is made on presentation. Surgical procedures for erectile dysfunction vary from penile revascularization to the insertion of prosthetic implants.

Answer 10

(a) Acute tubular necrosis
Acute rejection
Obstruction of the collecting system
Infarction of transplant 2

(b) Daily serum U&E
Isotope renography for state of perfusion
Ultrasonography – reveals urinary tract obstruction, haematoma, urinoma and renal artery flow
Percutaneous renal biopsy to diagnose acute tubular necrosis or acute rejection 3

		Marks
(c) (i)	Cyclosporin A and/or azathioprine, anti-thymocyte globulin and prednisolone	2
(ii)	Increased incidence of malignancies, i.e. with azathioprine immunosuppression, e.g. tumours of reticulo-endothelial system, central nervous system and skin Increased incidence of upper GI bleeding with high doses of steroids	2

Comment

Oliguria or anuria due to acute tubular necrosis occurs immediately post-transplantation, the extent of the tubular damage is dependent on the warm ischaemia time of the donor kidney. Dialysis must be continued until the kidney recovers. Rejection of the donor organ may be acute (within three months) or chronic (thereafter), with progressive impairment of urine production. The former responds favourably to anti-rejection therapy.

Answer 11

(a) (i)	Pelvi-ureteric colic due to renal calculus disease	1
(ii)	Test urine for red blood cells	2
(b)	Adequate analgesia Plain abdominal X-ray (KUB) and IVU to establish site of calculus If calculus is <5 mm in size await spontaneous passage If calculus is >5 mm in size cystoscopic basket extraction If impacted in intravesical portion of distal ureter, cysto-ureterotomy Shock-wave lithotripsy or operative removal may be indicated for stones in the renal pelvis and proximal ureter	5
(c)	Hereditary and acquired defects in calcium and phosphate metabolism Hyperparathyroidism	

Hyperoxaluria **Marks**
Cystinuria 2

Comment

The need for open surgery for renal stones has been largely replaced by endoscopic or percutaneous extraction and by extracorporeal shock-wave lithotripsy. Ureteric catheterization and irrigation frequently dislodges impacted uteric calculi; occasionally those impacted above the pelvic brim may be pushed up into the renal pelvis and fragmented or extracted percutaneously. Leaking abdominal aneurysms may mimic left-sided renal colic and are rapidly fatal unless promptly resuscitated and operated upon.

Answer 12

(a) (i) Hydronephrosis
Cystic kidney
Nephroblastoma (Wilms' tumour)
Mesoblastic nephroma 2

(ii) Ultrasound
CT and/or MRI scans of the abdomen
IVU
Renal angiography 3

(b) (i) CXR
Liver scan
Bone scan
Bone marrow biopsy 2

(ii) Surgical: Radical nephroureterectomy

Radiotherapy: Pre- and/or post-operative courses

Chemotherapy: Childhood tumours of the kidney or adjacent neuroectoderm are chemosensitive and respond well to a combination of two or more agents 3

Comment **Marks**

Nephroblastomas and neuroblastomas usually present as palpable loin swellings and anaemia. Both lesions, as well as the rarer mesoblastoma of the kidney, require radical excision. Radiotherapy may be given prior to surgery to reduce the tumour bulk, and a post-operative course is usual. Chemotherapy is usually a combination of actinomycin D and vincristine or cyclophosphamide and doxorubicin or cisplatin.

Answer 13

(a) Urethral stricture

Inflammatory – chronic urethritis (e.g. venereal infection)
Traumatic – perineal injury producing partial rupture or ischaemic damage
Iatrogenic – following urethral instrumentation or prostatic surgery in the older male 3

(b) Urinary retention leads to bladder diverticulae, hydroureter and hydronephrosis
Proximal urethral diverticulum leads to periurethral abscess and urethral fisulae (watering can perineum)
Increased abdominal pressure of straining gives rise to groin herniae, piles and rectal prolapse 3

(c) Intermittent urethral dilatation with gum-elastic bougies, either separate or filiform with screw-on followers
Self-dilatation with soft Nelaton catheters

Urethrotomy under direct vision using an optical urethrotome

Urethroplasty by excision of stricture and end-to-end anastomosis or grafting following excision of more extensive strictures 4

Comment

Gonococcal urethritis must be actively treated with antibiotics, with the prevention of re-exposure. Ineffective treatment may lead to spread of infection to produce posterior urethritis, prostatitis, epididymo-orchitis or periurethral abscess. Dilatation of urethral strictures may introduce infection resulting in a bacteraemia and/or septicaemia; aseptic technique is, therefore, essential. **Marks**

Answer 14

(a) Stress incontinence is caused by sphincter weakness and produces urinary leakage as a result of increased intra-abdominal pressure

Causes: Weakness of distal sphincter mechanism combined with laxity of pelvic floor musculature due to complicated or neglected labour or multiple pregnancies

Neurogenic bladder dysfunction due to demyelinating diseases (myelodysplasia, multiple sclerosis, syringomyelia) 3

(b) Exercise testing with 300 ml of fluid in bladder and measure resulting fluid loss (in the order of 10–50 ml)
Pressure–flow studies record bladder pressure and flow rate during micturition (distinguishes between genuine stress incontinence and detrusor instability) 2

(c) Minor degrees of stress incontinence can be controlled by improving the tone of the pelvic floor musculature by pelvic floor exercises
Surgical measures: colposuspension (suspending the vaginal fascia on either side of the bladder neck to the ileopubic ligaments)
Neurogenic bladder dysfunction may require implantation of a battery-operated urinary sphincter stimulator 4

Comment
It is important to distinguish stress incontinence from idiopathic detrusor muscle instability, as the outcome of surgery is significantly worse in the latter. The mainstay of treatment in the latter is the use of anticholinergic agents. Symptoms of stress incontinence due to neurogenic bladder dysfunction may progress to complete incontinence or to retention as the disease progresses.

CHAPTER 11: VASCULAR SURGERY

Answer 1 **Marks**

(a) Diagnosis: acute limb ischaemi due to left common femoral arterial occlusion

Predisposing factors:
Atrial fibrillation leading to embolism
Thrombus on a previously diseased artery
Aortic dissection 3

(b) Pallor and/or skin mottling
Cold, pulselessness and pain
Reduced skin sensation
Loss of function (toes cannot be moved)
Venous guttering 3

(c) Emergency surgical work-up:
FBC, U&E, CXR, ECG, urethral catheterization
Group and cross-match 4 units

Treat as acute or acute-on-chronic occlusion with systemic anticoagulation, aterial embolectomy or thrombectomy, with per-operative angiogram
In some instances thromboembolytic therapy may avoid surgery 4

Comment
Acute limb ischaemia is a surgical emergency. Systemic heparinization (35,000–45,000 units per 24 hr) is commenced, and thrombo-embolectomy performed with a Fogarty balloon catheters. Occasionally, thrombolysis may be achieved with fibrinolytic agents, such as streptokinase or tissue plasminogen activator (tPA), which is infused intra-arterially. Long-term warfarin therapy must be commenced or the precipitating cause treated to prevent recurrence.

Answer 2

(a) (i) Peripheral vascular disease producing stenosis of the arteries of the right lower limb

	Marks
Right common femoral artery or superficial and profunda femoral arteries	2
(ii) Pathogenesis of atherosclerosis: adherent microthrombi and subintimal cholesterol deposits lead to atheromatous plaque formation and luminal narrowing; plaque haemorrhage leads to intimal ulceration; thrombi form on the ulcerated surface, giving rise to microemboli producing distal vessel occlusion	3
(b) Smoking Diabetes mellitus Hypercholesterolaemia/high fat intake Hypertension Family history	2
(c) Stop smoking Close monitoring of diabetes/hypertension and response to treatment Exercise to develop collateral circulation, weight reduction, low cholesterol diet Foot care: chiropody, protective footwear	3

Comment

Claudication can usually be distinguished from musculo-skeletal symptoms in the lower limb from the history of exercise-related pain. Peripheral vascular disease is generalized in nature, and the carotid arteries and the aorta must be clinically assessed for occult lesions. The nutritional state of the affected foot, namely skin changes and brachial–ankle pressure indices, form part of the initial assessment.

Answer 3

(a) Pale, cold limb with loss of sensation, ischaemic skin changes Reduced or absent femoral, popliteal, dorsalis pedis, posterior tibial Reduced ankle–brachial pressure indices Neurological signs: Reduced sensation, tone, power and reflexes with muscle wasting	4

		Marks
(b)	(i) Retrograde transfemoral aortography	1
	(ii) Angioplasty of stenotic arterial lesions Intra-arterial infusion of tissue plasmin activator (tPA) at the site of stenosis through a radiologically positioned arterial catheter	2
(c)	Removal of arterial occlusive disease by endarterectomy Bypass of occlusion using native vein or synthetic vascular grafts	3

Comment

The presence of rest pain and brachial–ankle pressure index of >0.5 suggest critical ischaemia. Pain usually involve the leg and foot, and there may be sensory or motor signs. Vascular reconstruction is usually required for limb salvage. However, in the presence of distal vessel disease, unresponsive to angioplasty or surgery, lumbar sympathectomy may improve skin perfusion.

Answer 4

(a)	Claudication or rest pain extending up to the buttock Weak or absent distal pulses Low resting and exercise brachial–ankle pressure indices Loss of muscle power	3
(b)	(i) Thrombosis, dislodgement of atheromatous plaque, or intimal dissection during or following angioplasty producing arterial occlusion	2
	(ii) Analgesia; anticoagulation with IV heparin Infusion of prostaglandin-derived thrombolytic agent (tPA) Thrombo-embolectomy; repair or removal of intimal flap	3
(c)	Smoking Diabetes mellitus Hyperlipidaemia/high fat intake Hypertension Family history	2

Comment **Marks**

Vascular imaging and interventional procedures are common in cardiology and vascular units. Complications arising therefrom, though uncommon, may require urgent surgical intervention. Patients who are admitted for these procedures must, therefore, be adequately assessed and prepared with informed consent for such eventualities.

Answer 5

			Marks
(a)	(i)	False aneurysm of femoral artery	1
	(ii)	Duplex Doppler scan	1
	(iii)	By pressure occlusion or, failing this, by surgical repair of arterial wall defect	2
(b)	(i)	Thrombosis, embolus, intimal plaque formation, intimal dissection	2
	(ii)	Embolectomy/thrombectomy under imaging; intimal repair	4

Comment

A false aneurysm is a pulsatile haematoma produced by bleeding from the arterial puncture. Rarely, the adjacent femoral vein may be injured, with the formation of a traumatic arteriovenous fistula. This also presents as a pulsatile groin swelling. If detected early the fistula may be closed off by pressure occlusion with a Doppler probe. If allowed to mature it requires surgical repair. Fibrinolytic therapy may lead to recanalization following angiographic assessment of the site of thrombotic arterial occlusion.

Answer 6

			Marks
(a)	(i)	Abdominal aortic aneurysm	1
	(ii)	Atherosclerotic changes to vessel wall with intimal ulceration and destruction of elastic and muscle coats with intraluminal thrombus formation	2

Marks

(b) Abdominal ultrasound scan 1

(c) (i) Aneurysms <6 cm in diameter and asymptomatic – keep under surveillance
Aneurysms >6 cm in diameter – inlay of synthetic graft 3

(ii) Pre-operative work-up:
CXR, FBC
ECG
Renal function assessment
Hypertension control

Group and cross-match 6–8 units of blood 3

Comment
Abdominal aneurysms over 6 cm in diameter expand progressively over time, increasing the incidence of rupture or leakage. Elective surgery is aimed at obviating this risk, as survival following rupture is small. The chances of dying from rupture of aneurysms <6 cm are the same as dying from elective aneurysectomy, therefore a conservative approach is followed, provided the patient is kept under surveillance. Image-guided intra-luminal grafting of aneurysms is being assessed and may obviate the need for open surgery.

Answer 7

(a) (i) Rupture of abdominal aortic aneurysm 1

(ii) Resuscitation:
Maintain airway, administer O_2
Central and peripheral venous access
FBC and ABG
IV analgesia
Group and emergency cross-match for 10–15 units of blood
Monitor pulse, BP and respiration quarter-hourly
Volume replacement with crystalloids and plasma expanders, and with blood when available

	Marks
Catheterize and monitor urine output Inform the surgical and anaesthetic teams and the theatre in preparation for emergency surgery CXR, AXR and ECG (if time permits) Consent patient for emergency abdominal surgery	3
(b) Aneurysectomy and Dacron graft repair of ruptured aortic aneurysm	1
(c) (i) Spontaneous retroperitoneal haemorrhage due to over-anticoagulation	2
(ii) i.v. analgesia Stop warfarin therapy Resuscitation and replace blood volume Administer coagulation factors in the form of fresh frozen plasma and platelet concentrates	3

Comment

It is vital to distinguish on presentation from a ruptured or leaking aneurysm left-sided pelvi-ureteric colic or diverticulitis of the left colon. Occasionally, retrosternal radiation of pain, coupled with circulatory collapse may simulate myocardial infarction. A pulsatile and expansile abdominal mass and weak or absent femoral pulses must be sought on examining the abdomen. Surgical survival is determined largely by the duration of hypotension (the interval between rupture and surgical control), this determines the incidence of cardio-respiratory complications and coagulation disorders in the post-operative period.

Answer 8

(a) (i) Stenosis of the right internal carotid artery	1
(ii) Hypertension, diabetes mellitus, smoking, hyperlipidaemia, family history	2
(b) (i) Bilateral carotid angiography	1

Marks

(ii) Site and extent of atheromatous disease of the carotid and intracranial arteries, and cross-perfusion between the two hemispheres 2

(c) Treat pre-existing cardiac disease and/or hypertension; control diabetes mellitus
Treat hyperlipidaemia
Right carotid endarterectomy
Post-operatively systolic pressure to be kept below 100 mmHg 4

Comment

Atherosclerotic narrowing or ulceration is generally widespread despite symptoms being confined to one anatomic region, supplied by one or more diseased vessels. There is, therefore, the need to assess the contralateral carotid supply, myocardial and renal function, and the presence of other risk factors for stroke before planning surgery.

Answer 9

(a) Venous and vasculitic ulcers are caused by skin breakdown, due to poor nutrition
Venous bleeding follows the erosion of the ulcer into an adjacent or underlying varicosity 3

(b) Tourniquets are to be avoided in first aid as they cause venous congestion and increased blood loss; they cause arterial damage if applied too tightly
Venous haemorrhage is readily controlled by elevation of the affected limb and a pressure dressing 3

(c) Control local oedema by graduated support stockings or limb elevation
Appropriate topical ulcer treatment until healing is complete
Surgical removal of the underlying varices 4

Comment **Marks**

Tourniquets can cause exsanguination by preventing venous outflow but not arterial inflow. Tourniquets tight enough to occlude the latter may cause vascular damage and thrombosis. Nerve conduction injury may also occur and, if applied for a number of hours, may produce muscle necrosis and precipitate renal failure. Arterial tourniquet is used for some surgical procedures, but should not be left in place for more than an hour.

Answer 10

(a) (i) Venous or stasis ulcer caused by trophic skin changes and underlying venous stasis — 1

(ii) Indolent, shallow and moist granulating floor with associated varicosities and surrounding pigmentation
Induration and pitting oedema leads to poor skin nutrition — 2

(b) (i) Limb elevation; daily wound toilet and non-stick dressing
Split-skin grafting if required — 2

(ii) Treat the associated varicose veins surgically following ulcer healing — 1

(c) Ischaemic ulcers: caused by poor tissue perfusion due to pressure (decubitus ulcers), atherosclerotic or diabetic vascular occlusive disease
Neuropathic ulcers are anaesthetic and are caused by peripheral nerve degeneration, as in leprosy and diabetic neuritis
Tropical ulcers are due to chronic skin infections caused by bacteria (*Mycobacterium ulcerans* in Buruli ulcer) or fungi (actinomycosis, mycetoma) — 4

Comment

Ulcers due to vascular diseases are painful; the exceptions being pressure ulcers and diabetic ulcers where nerve damage occurs alongside the ischaemic changes.

Venous ulcers in the leg may extend and become circumferential, thereby endangering the viability of the limb. Chronicity may give rise to squamous cell carcinoma (Marjolin's ulcer); biopsy should be undertaken when in doubt. **Marks**

Answer 11

(a) Increase in body temperature and pulse
Increase in limb diameter and warmth
Tenderness on palpation, with or without induration
Postive Homans' sign 3

(b) (i) Deep vein thrombosis (DVT) of calf and/or thigh 1

(ii) Venous stasis leads to the following sequence: DVT, pulmonary embolus, fall in pulmonary arterial pressure, with consequent fall in gaseous exchange, fall in cardiac output and cardiac arrest 3

(c) Management of DVT:
Colour flow duplex imaging confirms DVT and its proximal extent. (Venogram gives further information on the iliac veins.)
IV heparin infusion of 30,000–40,000 IU/24 hr
Commence long-term warfarin therapy before discharge; monitor anticoagulation profile periodically 3

Comment

In young patients, in addition to known risk factors, such as oral contraception and smoking, spontaneous venous thrombosis may be associated with deficiencies in the coagulation profile, i.e. protein C, protein S and antithrombin III. Prolonged immobility in healthy adults, as in long-haul flights, may predispose to DVT. Thrombosis of the common femoral vein with an associated lymphangitis produces a very swollen 'white leg' (phlegmasia alba dolens); extensive thrombosis of the iliac and pelvic veins produces venous obstruction and a 'blue leg' (phlegmasia caerulea dolens). In the latter, venous gangrene may threaten limb viability.

Answer 12 **Marks**

(a) (i) Pulmonary embolus 1

(ii) ECG
Ventilation/perfusion scan
ABG 2

(b) Resuscitation
Analgesia
Systemic anticoagulation
Swan–Ganz catheterization to measure pulmonary artery wedge pressure and for selective thrombolysis
Surgical embolectomy if cardiorespiratory function deteriorates 5

(c) Stop smoking; avoid oral contraception
Compression stockings
Early mobilization
Heparin prophylaxis 2

Comment

Pulmonary emboli originate from thrombus in the veins of the pelvis or lower limbs. The latter may give rise to local symptoms and/or signs and signal an impending catastrophe. Deep venous thrombosis must, therefore, be actively treated with immediate systemic anticoagulation. Thrombosis in pelvic veins extending to the inferior vena cava may require angiographic placement of a filter above it to prevent embolization.

SECTION III:
ESSAY WRITING

CHAPTER 1: STRUCTURED OUTLINES

QUESTION 1

Write an essay on the diagnosis and treatment of primary skin cancers.

Plan

Types of skin cancer:
- Rodent cancer
- Melanoma
- Squamous cell carcinoma
- Kaposi's sarcoma

Initiating factors (if any)

Diagnosis:
- History – duration, scabbing/bleeding, pain, etc.
- Site and size
- Appearance – surface, edges, base
- Histology
- Regional lymphadenopathy

Treatment:
- Surgical – wide local excision (except Kaposi's)
- Block dissection of involved regional nodes
- Adjuvant – radio-, chemo-, immunotherapies

Prognosis:
- Dependent on type, histological grading and spread (nodal/visceral)

Follow-up:
- Long term for all except rodent ulcers
- Treatment of recurrences

QUESTION 2

Write an essay on the management of a 36-year-old man who sustained a spinal injury at C7–T1 level in a riding accident.

Plan

Immediate measures:
- Primary survey:
  - airway maintenance
  - BP, pulse and respiratory monitoring
  - neurological assessment
  - resuscitation
- Secondary survey:
  - detailed physical examination

Assessment of injuries:
- Neurological deficits
- Associated injuries

Treatment:
- Surgical – stabilize spinal fracture/dislocation
- Supportive – maintenance of bodily function:
  - nutrition
  - bladder
  - bowel
- Monitor recovery of neurological function
- Avoid morbidity: viz, bed sores, bone demineralization, muscle atrophy
- Physiotherapy – maximize functional recovery by exercise regimes and physical aids
- Community care – adjustments to home/work environment
- Long-term complications of paraplegia

QUESTION 3

A 30-year-old woman presents with an asymptomatic lump in her left breast. Discuss your clinical assessment and management.

Plan

Working diagnosis on history and clinical features

Investigations:
- Mammogram/ultrasound scan
- FNAB
- Biopsy (excisional/incisional)
- Further investigations, e.g. CXR, bone and liver scans, if indicated

Definitive diagnosis from above

Counselling of patient

Treatment:
- Surgical:
  - benign – local excision
  - malignant – mastectomy (segmental or total)
  - axillary dissection
- Adjuvant therapy:
  - based on histological type and spread:
  - regional DXT
  - tamoxifen
  - chemotherapy
  - endocrine ablation (oophorectomy, adrenalectomy, hypophysectomy)

Follow up:
- Long term (annual after five years' recurrence-free)
- Diagnosis, re-staging and treatment of recurrent disease

QUESTION 4

Write an essay on the causes, presentation and treatment of obstructive jaundice.

Plan

Causes:

Congenital – biliary atresia
Inflammatory – sclerosing cholangitis
Infective – ascending cholangitis; parasitic (round) worms
Metabolic – duct stones or sludge
Iatrogenic – bile duct injury
Neoplastic – cholangiocarcinoma; periampulatory carcinoma, metatastic spread to lymph nodes in portahepatitis

Presentation:

Symptoms – weakness, loss of appetite, fever, itchiness, pale stools
Signs – jaundice, hepatomegaly, ascites, palpable gall bladder

Treatment:

Relief of obstruction:
By percutaneous trans-hepatic drainage and cholangiogram and/or ERCP to identify lesion
Antibiotic therapy on bile culture
Surgical measures:
Duct exploration, resection, biliary bypass
Endoscopic stenting with/without chemotherapy for inoperable lesions

QUESTION 5

Write an essay on the causation and the diagnosis of blood in the urine in a 70-year-old man.

Plan

Causes:
- Kidneys – acute nephritis, stone, tumour
- Ureter – stone, tumour
- Bladder – acute cystitis, polyps, tumour, stone (schistosomiasis)
- Prostate – tumour, prostatic surgery
- Urethra – stone
- Unknown aetiology

History:
- Duration of haematuria
- Blood mixed in urine or appears at start/end of micturition
- Stranguary
- Abdominal symptoms, if any

Clinical findings:
- General – pallor, BP, pulse
- Renal/bladder mass
- Prostatic enlargement
- Urethral lesion

Investigations:
- FBC, U&E
- MSU to confirm haematuria and to test for sugar
- Ultrasound scan of kidneys/bladder
- IVU
- If the above are negative/normal – repeat urinary microscopy
- If haematuria persists – uteric catherization for selective urine samples
- Renal imaging
- Once lesion is identified – histological confirmation by endoscopic biopsy or FNAB under imaging

QUESTION 6

Write an essay on the causation, presentation and treatment of small bowel obstruction.

Plan

Causes:

Intraluminal – bolus obstruction

In bowel wall – lymphoid hyperplasia and tumours leading to intussusception, vascular occulsion (mesenteric infarction)

Extraneous – internal herniations; external hernias

Iatrogenic – surgical adhesions or incisional herniae

Presentation:

Symptoms and signs of complete/incomplete obstruction, viz vomiting, dehydration, constipation, colic, abdominal signs

Characteristics of palpable mass or visible peristalsis

Signs of bowel ischaemia

AXR – erect and supine:

Air–fluid levels, level of obstruction from the configuration of proximal distended loops

Treatment:

Nasogastric suction

Rehydrate, electrolyte replacement

Urgent surgical relief of obstruction, except in adhesion obstruction when non-surgical measures are continued

Repair of causative hernia at same time

CHAPTER 2: MODEL ESSAYS

QUESTION:

Write an essay on the presentation and management of chronic arterial disease of the lower limb.

ANSWER 1 – A COMFORTABLE PASS

Introduction

Chronic arterial disease afflicting the aorta, the iliacs and vessels in the lower limb may produce stenosis, occlusion or aneurysmal dilatation. Atherosclerosis is the common vascular lesion and may also involve coronary, cerebral and renal arteries. Association risk factors are diabetes mellitus, hypertension, smoking, raised blood lipid levels and a family history of vascular disease.

Symptoms and signs

Stenosis of the main arteries reduces the blood flow to the lower limb producing intermittent claudication due to temporary muscle ischaemia: the claudication distance is the distance the patient is able to walk before stopping. Rest pain in the limb indicates severe restriction to blood flow, which is inadequate for resting tissue metabolism. The pain is characteristically in the foot, worse at night and relieved by dangling the limb out of bed or sleeping in a chair. Pain referred to the limb from degenerative disease of the lumbo-sacral spine, the hip or the knee or due to peripheral neuropathy must be distinguished from ischaemic pain.

Coldness, numbness and paraesthesia are present with skin pallor on elevating and duskiness on lowering the limb. Buerger's angle is the angle of elevation at which blanching first occurs and is accompanied by venous emptying or, in severe ischaemia, venous guttering. The time taken for the veins to refill on hanging the limb down indicates the extent of vascular compromise. In severe ischaemia the skin may be mottled and without sensation. Occasionally, symptoms and signs of acute-on-chronic ischaemia develop.

Ulceration occurs with severe arterial insufficiency and presents as painful, indolent, non-healing ulcers in the toes or pressure areas in the foot and occasionally over the ankle or the shin. Arterial pulses are reduced or absent distal to the diseased artery and occasionally a thrill or a bruit may be detected over the latter, caused by turbulent flow.

The presence of a pulsatile and expansile swelling in the abdomen indicates an aortic aneurysm, whereas a femoral or a popliteal aneurysm may be felt in the groin or behind the knee. They may be asymptomatic but can present with acute rupture or thrombosis.

Investigations

The severity of the symptoms determines the need for vascular investigations, and non-invasive ultrasound tests are performed routinely on presentation. The ankle–brachial pressure index is the ratio of systolic pressure in the ankle to that in the arm. The normal is 1.0. In claudicants the resting index is usually <1.0 and falls below the resting value following exercise. A resting index of ≤0.5 indicates critical ischaemia. The results of non-invasive tests indicate the need for further assessment with a view to treatment. Angiography by conventional or digital techniques demonstrates the anatomical site or sites and the severity of the disease process and enables treatment to be planned.

Treatment

Most claudicants require only reassurance and advice regarding weight reduction, low fat diet and stopping smoking, as appropriate. Intercurrent diseases, such as diabetes and hypertension, must be actively treated. Daily exercise regimes to improve the blood supply by developing collateral circulations must be actively encouraged. Foot care is essential to avoid injury to skin that may already be compromised. A daily aspirin tablet (75 mg) improves tissue perfusion by lowering the blood viscoscity.

In the presence of incapacitating claudication or rest pain, transluminal angioplasty is used as the first line of treatment. It dilates the stenosed lumen with an inflatable balloon introduced on an arterial catheter under fluoroscopic screening. Intraluminal stents may occasionally be inserted to keep the lumen open following dilatation.

Surgery for occlusive disease is indicated when angioplasty is not feasible. Aortic or aorto–iliac disease may be bypassed with a Dacron tube or bifurcation graft; in the case of aortic or iliac aneurysm the sac is opened and the graft sutured in. When intra-abdominal surgery is contraindicated, grafts are placed from the ipsilateral axillary or the contralateral common femoral arteries.

Arterial narrowing below the inguinal ligament is bypassed using the long saphenous vein. In its absence a PTFA graft is used and to prolong its patency a collar of vein is interposed between the distal end of the graft and the recipient artery. Aneurysms in the limb are similarly bypassed and are excluded from the circulation to prevent emboli from the clot present within them. Skin perfusion may be improved by lumbar sympathectomy when revascularisation is not feasible.

Clinical and sonographic surveillance is important in monitoring graft patency and impending graft occlusion. With progressive deterioration in symptoms, amputation of the limb should be considered with a planned rehabilitation programme aimed at restoring mobility. This includes physiotherapy and involvement of occupational therapists to ensure that home conditions are appropriate for discharge from hospital.

Examiner's Comments on Answer 1

- *The essay is eminently readable, knowledgeable and concise, with appropriate subdivisions*
- *The introduction defines the problem, gives emphasis to atherosclerosis with its risk factors*
- *Diagnosis is based on the history, examination and investigations, and the candidate has commented on the relevant points in each group*
- *The question is very broad and, therefore, treatment can only be covered in outline. Clear guidelines on each treatment modality are stated*
- *Emphasis is given to the conservative management of most patients, and medical management available is outlined*
- *The importance of angioplasty is given as the first line of management, and the main forms of surgical intervention are summarised*
- *The importance of follow-up is stated*
- *The possible need for amputation is noted, together with the necessary team work for subsequent rehabilitation*

ANSWER 2 – AN ANSWER SHOWING INADEQUATE KNOWLEDGE

The aetiology of chronic arterial disease of the lower limbs is poor general health due to various organic disease states and poor lifestyle. Presentation may be divided into symptoms and signs. The classic symptom of chronic arterial disease of the lower limb is pain. This may be constant or intermittent, and described as affecting mainly the feet or the entire limb, but the most usual presentation is intermittent claudication, this being a sharp pain affecting one or both calves that is induced by exercise and relieved by rest. It is often more troublesome in cold weather. The amount of exercise necessary to bring on the pain is extremely variable but the most troublesome confounding factor in eliciting a history of claudication is the co-existence of osteoarthritis which may make exercise painful and may even mask the presence of arterial disease by precluding walking on its own account. Pain may also arise as a result of ulceration and the patient may complain of cold legs. In late-stage disease a blackened toe may be the presentation. Whilst pain is a feature of ischaemia, tissue which has died is anaesthetic, manipulation of areas of gangrene may cause severe pain at the granulating demarcation between living and dead tissue. Patients with chronic disease may occasionally present acutely, either with a complete cessation of blood flow secondary to thrombus formation, leading to paralysis of the limb which becomes pale, paraesthetic and cold with undetectable pulses or with life-threatening gas gangrene where the patient is systemically ill and the offending limb is pale or green, malodorous and may exhibit the characteristic 'crackling' sensation of gas in the tissues on examination.

Signs of chronic arterial disease of the lower limb include loss of hair, cool skin, ulcers that are characteristically small and well-demarcated, pulses which are difficult or impossible to palpate, blackened extremities and stumps which are sites of previous amputations. The femoral pulses ought always to be auscultated as bruits will often be heard. The management of chronic arterial disease may be divided into investigations, medical and surgical treatment, nursing and physiotherapy. Various radiological investigations may be performed. Such investigations may include angiography, whereas MRI (magnetic resonance imaging) may make a big impact on angiography in the future by allowing digital subtraction images to be constructed non-invasively. Medical treatment will almost always include an anti-clotting agent, such as aspirin, typically 75 mg once daily. Treatment of co-existing medical illness, particularly coronary artery disease should not be overlooked. A number of drugs are available to promote arterial dilation in the peripheries.

Surgical intervention may include endarterectomy if the lesion is relatively localized and in an accessible position. Bypass grafts using PTFE tubing are most useful for restoring blood supply. They may be done at various levels and the femoral–popliteal graft is the classic operation. Surgical treatment often involves amputation if conservative treatment of areas of gangrenous tissue fails. Amputation requires a balance between leaving as much viable tissue as possible and ensuring that the tissue left remains viable; patients are often medically so ill that re-operation is even more undesirable than usual. Nursing care includes care of the whole patient, dressing of ulcers and scrupulous attention to hygiene on areas of tissue which may have died or are of dubious viability. Physiotherapy may improve the function of existing limbs and aid familiarization with artificial limbs, crutches, etc.

Examiner's Comments on Answer 2

Reads well, with many common sense statements, but:

- *Introduction limited to a vague statement, with no mention of risk factors*
- *No sub-headings*
- *Inadquate paragraphs*
- *Too much emphasis given to osteoarthritis and gas gangrene, which have little relevance to the question set*
- *Pain affects the 'entire limb'*
- *Nutrition and postural changes in the foot are missing*
- *No mention of non-invasive tests, viz pressure measurements, imaging or wave-form analysis*
- *No mention of indications for angiography*
- *No mention of drugs, such as anti-platelet agents and their limitations, and PTA – the current first choice of therapeutic measure*
- *No mention of aorto-iliac disease*
- *No mention of extra-anatomic bypass or the limitations of synthetic grafts across the knee*
- *The importance of amputations was mentioned, but no occupational therapy or rehabilitation of the amputee*

SECTION IV:
ESSAY QUESTIONS

ESSAY QUESTIONS

SURGICAL PHYSIOLOGY

1. Discuss the principles of post-operative fluid and electrolyte balance.

2. Describe the preparation of a patient for an abdominal operation and the immediate post-operative management.

3. What is meant by circulatory collapse and shock? List the causes and describe how you would treat one of them.

4. Discuss the investigation and management of a patient who is alleged to have a 'bleeding tendency' before and after major surgery.

TRAUMA AND BURNS

1. A 14-year-old boy is admitted to the Accident and Emergency department with a right-sided abdominal pain after falling 15 feet from a tree. Discuss your assessment and treatment.

2. Describe the priorities of diagnosis and management in a severely injured person.

3. A 10-year-old girl lacerated her wrist on a plate glass window. Describe the structures that may be damaged, indicating how such damage may be diagnosed and treated.

4. Write an essay on the management of skin burns.

5. Discuss the management of a 23-year-old man who was crushed when the seating terrace collapsed at a football stadium.

ORTHOPAEDICS

1. Discuss the management of a 67-year-old woman with osteoarthritis of the hip.

2. A young man was seen in the Orthopaedic clinic with a painful swollen knee following a rotational football injury three days before. Discuss the diagnosis and outline your management.

3. Describe the management and potential complications in a 65-year-old woman with a compound fracture of the tibia and fibula.

4. Write an essay on the diagnosis and treatment of fractures of the femur in an adult.

5. An 80-year-old woman complains of pain in her thoracic spine. Discuss the differential diagnoses and the management of the commonest cause of such a symptom.

NEUROSURGERY

1. Write an essay on the assessment and treatment of an adult patient admitted unconscious following a road traffic accident.

2. Describe the various types of peripheral nerve injuries and how you would evaluate and treat them.

3. Describe the common forms of spina bifida and discuss its complications and treatment.

   or

   Write an essay on hydrocephalus and its management.

EYES, ENT AND SKIN

1. Discuss the diagnosis and management of a 36-year-old woman with a malignant melanoma of the skin over her calf.

2. A young man presents to the Accident and Emergency department with discomfort and hazy vision in one eye a few hours after working with a hammer and chisel. What are the possible findings? Discuss the investigations and treatment that may be indicated.

3. Discuss the clinical presentation, the complications and treatment of chronic suppurative otitis media.

4. Describe the causes of a painful red eye and the management of this condition.

5. Describe the causes and discuss the management of a patient with severe nose bleed.

ENDOCRINOLOGY, BREAST AND CHEST

1. Write an essay on the disorders that may arise from abnormalities of the adrenal glands and their surgical treatment.

2. Describe the diagnosis and management of a 40-year-old woman who presents with a solitary nodule in the left lobe of the thyroid.

3. Discuss the diagnosis and management of a 35-year-old woman presenting with a painless lump in the breast.

4. List the causes and discuss the diagnosis and management of a patient with a pneumothorax.

5. Write an essay on the presentation, aetiology, investigation and treatment of a carcinoma of the bronchus.

6. Write an essay on the investigation and interventional and surgical measures used in treating ischaemic heart disease.

UPPER ALIMENTARY TRACT

1. A 64-year-old man presents with a three-month history of increasing difficulty in swallowing solid food. Discuss the diagnosis and management of this patient.

2. Write an essay on the diagnosis and treatment of haematemesis in a 56-year-old woman.

3. Discuss the surgical causes of vomiting in a 14-day-old neonate. Describe how you would diagnose and treat one such condition.

4. Discuss the diagnosis and management of a patient with a perforated peptic ulcer.

5. Write an essay on the indications for splenectomy and the complications of this procedure.

LIVER, GALLBLADDER AND PANCREAS

1. Write an essay on the diagnosis and treatment of a patient suffering from acute cholecystitis.

2. Discuss the presentation, the diagnosis and management of a 68-year-old man with obstructive jaundice.

3. Write an essay on the aetiology, diagnosis and management of acute pancreatitis.

4. Write an essay on portal hypertension and its management.

5. Discuss the causes of liver abscess and its treatment.

SMALL AND LARGE BOWEL

1. Discuss the aetiology and complications of diverticulitis of the colon. Describe the clinical features of the disease and the principles of treatment.

2. Discuss the diagnosis and management of a 32-year-old man who presents with a painful, tender mass in the right iliac fossa.

3. Write an essay on the differential diagnosis and management of a 65-year-old woman complaining of left lower abdominal pain and constipation of 10 weeks' duration.

4. An 18-month-old boy said to be suffering from abdominal colic passed bloodstained mucus per rectum. Discuss the diagnosis and management.

UROLOGY

1. A 35-year-old man presented to the Surgical clinic with a hard, painless swelling of the scrotum. Describe the management of this patient.

2. Describe the management of an adult presenting with haematuria.

3. Describe the types of undescended testis, its treatment and complications.

4. Describe the clinical presentation and management of a patient with a hypernephroma (Grawitz tumour).

5. Write an essay on urethral stricture in an adult male.

VASCULAR SURGERY

1. Describe the causes, presentation and management of an embolus of the femoral artery in a 50-year-old woman seen within six hours of the onset of symptoms.

2. A 61-year-old man presents to the Surgical clinic with a nine-month history of pain in his right calf that occurs after walking 100 yards on the flat, and is relieved by rest. Discuss the diagnosis and management of this patient and the factors that would influence the latter.

3. Discuss the causes and describe the management of gangrene of the toes.

4. Discuss the management of a 70-year-old man presenting with an asymptomatic, pulsatile and expansile mass in the abdomen.

5. Discuss the aetiology and management of lower leg ulceration.

APPENDIX A:
THE FINAL EXAMINATION IN SURGERY

Assessment of clinical competence

Medical training encompasses a wide range of complex and varied activities and has evolved to match the diverse abilities required of the practising clinician. Maintaining these skills is essential for the establishment of professional standards of excellence and satisfying public expectation.

Assessment of clinical competence over such a broad field is fraught with difficulty: it has to examine the results of a number of years of study, covering a large syllabus in a uniform, efficient, competent and reliable fashion. It should ensure that candidates who have achieved the required level of proficiency pass, and those who have not should fail. The examination should be seen by students and examiners as being fair.

The perfect examination not only has to accurately assess knowledge and understanding but also has to evaluate the powers of analysis in problem-solving and decision-making. In the clinical field the candidate's attitude to patients and clinical work, as well as their personal and professional development and conduct, must also be evaluated.

Why examine?

Over the last few decades a number of groups have questioned the need for formal assessment and have proposed continuous, faculty-based evaluation in medical education. Nevertheless, the vast majority of medical schools and universities rely on staged examinations to ensure the acquisition of a minimal knowledge base. Satisfactory performance may be accompanied by graduation, certification, and the right to practise. The level of achievement may influence progress and promotion.

Examinations are also valuable for students and teachers to establish personal and departmental standards, and one of the problems of statutory examinations is usually their lack of feedback of the details of a candidate's performance. Internal faculty examinations can be an aid to learning and a means of self-evlauation: this will become of increasing importance with the extension of continued medical education, to help students identify a weakness of personal knowledge and of teaching material. Even the most ardent supporters of continuous assessment cannot deny the stimulus and motivation of an examination, and it does separate good from bad candidates.

What system?

To justify their existence examinations have to be seen as fair and linked with both the training and its stated objectives. Traditional medical examinations have been based on the essay, the oral and the clinical. History and examination are central to a doctor–patient relationship, and the clinical has held its ground in undergraduate and postgraduate assessment (although the division between medicine, surgery and other disciplines has often become blurred, the emphasis being on the history and examination rather than the underlying disorder). Short cases in some schools have been replaced or supplemented by Objective Structured Clinical Examinations (OSCEs) to accompany the written part, and orals have been restricted to distinction and borderline candidates.

The essay has come under the greatest scrutiny. Students and examiners have questioned the effectiveness of an essay paper, since the limited number of topics and the possible choices have encouraged students to spot questions and concentrate on only part of the syllabus. The marking of essays is time-consuming and unreliable. There may be variation in the individual examiner's reassessment of papers, as well as between examiners. The variation makes comparison at a national level difficult, and this is further accentuated by what has been described as the deep psychological reluctance of examiners to allocate more than 70% of the total marks allowed for any given essay question.

Attempts to modify the essay included modified essay questions (MEQs), introducing a larger number of questions with a patient vignette, and a variety of sub-sections based on various aspects of diagnosis and treatment. Multiple short answers on a range of topics have also gained favour in some schools. Structured answer questions (SAQs) are a further development of the written assessment, testing problem-solving and decision-making in a structured and objective fashion. They are proving a reliable means of assessing knowledge and understanding in clinical practice.

MCQs also have a wide application in medical assessment, having the potential of covering a wide body of knowledge and, in their extended matching pairs format, introducing reasoned responses rather than item recall. A computerized marking system has eased the examiners' burden in this section. A current trend in the written part of the clinical examination is to include both MCQs and SAQs, the former to determine the candidate's knowledge, and the latter to assess the application of this knowledge by reasoning, interpretation, problem-solving and decision-making.

SAQs

SAQs test the candidate's high-level skills rather than factual recall. They consist of a clinical vignette followed by two to four questions, which may have sub-sections, with an indication of the marks allocated for each correct answer. The choice of scenario is based on common clinical problems pertinent and relevant to the field of study, and covering important concepts and principles relating to the course material. There is no room for trivia, irrelevant or esoteric topics, or interesting rarities.

Clinical information is presented in an ordered fashion, usually describing the history and examination, with or without investigations, of a specific condition. Questions should be clear, unambiguous and requiring the examinee to analyse and make decisions based on the given information. This may involve diagnosis or treatment and may also cover aspects of psychological, social and family history, and ethical issues.

Examiners are given a model answer and a marking schedule that has to be closely adhered to. Marking is time-consuming: allotting a single examiner to each question streamlines the process and allows uniformity of marking for a group of candidates. Any allowances made for near-misses will also be generalized. It is common to double mark a number of scripts to check examiners' inter-observer reliability across the whole examination.

Examiners preparing SAQs should form a panel, draw up a list of topics and allocate these topics among the group. The first draft of each question is read out at a group meeting, and comments made on the content, style, the importance, relevance, and its educational standard.

The second draft of the questions is tried on a group of students under examination conditions, noting the time taken to complete 4–8 questions.The answers are analysed and questions again modified if there are obvious misunderstandings, or unexpected ease or difficulty.

Misinterpretation of the stem may lead to an erroneous diagnosis. As the rest of the question is usually based on the stem, a candidate may go off at a tangent in all subsequent answers. The examiners must then make an informed decision in allocating marks for such mishaps, provided the conclusions reached are logical and not far-removed from the expected answers. However, in inadequately vetted questions more than one diagnosis may be arrived at from the stem. In such circumstances the onus is firmly on the examiner to accommodate such unanticipated correct responses and mark them fairly.

The completed questions are retained in a question bank. They should be added to each year, attention being given to the choice, number and range of topics. These should match the weighting given to each part of the syllabus. It may take three to five years to build up an adequate bank; after this time any break in security is of less importance.

The stem of a question can often be modified by changing the disease and superficial data, such as the sex, age and timing of the symptoms. This process eases the generation of further questions and allows some degree of comparison of standards when they are being analysed. Questions should be under continuous reappraisal after each use, to assess their performance and discriminatory value. Marks can be influenced by poor quality questions, poor knowledge of answers and errors within the marking system.

Each examination requires 10–12 questions to allow a broad assessment and to produce discriminatory differences between good and bad candidates. Each question used should be independent of the others.

Essays

MCQs are used routinely in most qualifying and postgraduate examinations. Nevertheless, medicine is not as black and white as MCQs would suggest, and many brighter students are adverse to this form of assessment. Similarly, although SAQs allow much wider coverage of the syllabus and more objectivity in the marking systems they also restrict the examiner to black or white rigid marking schemes. The limitations of these features are well-known to every clinician who has gone over recent examinations with groups of students.

The essay does test a candidate's ability to collect and quantify material, and assesses their powers of original thought and creativity. It determines the candidate's ability to write clear and legible English, and some schools have felt that these qualities should be retained in their assessment. In spite of the expensive manpower required in marking essay questions, an essay does assess a candidate's depth of knowledge in a specified area and, in preparing for an essay paper, candidates have to acquire detailed knowledge of much of the syllabus.

Revision for the essay paper is linked with revision of the whole course. If a candidate's knowledge base is poor, he or she will rightly fail; but, even if it is sound, good examination technique is essential for success. The ease of revision is based on previous knowledge and a good filing system which, if disease-based, provides a checklist for each condition so that current knowledge can be written and then checked against books and stored material to identify deficiencies.

The candidate is expected to have read around topics and patient problems encountered during the clinical course, gaining information from lectures, reviews, and current papers, as well as textbooks. This information should be filed in an easily retrievable form, such as notes in the margins of textbooks, a card system, plenty of lists and clearly written pieces of paper. People vary in the amount of information they can remember at any one time. Any deficiency, however, can be easily reversed during revision, provided previous information was well-organized and fully understood at the time it was collected.

Examiners at an undergraduate level are keen to pass candidates, to ensure that they can continue with their careers. However, medical examiners have an obligation to ensure that ignorant and potentially dangerous individuals are not let loose on a patient population. At a postgraduate level examiners have to ensure that a candidate has a comprehensive and in-depth knowledge of their subject: gaps are likely to be penalised.

Regardless of the level of the examination, essays on clinical subjects have a similar format. This is based on a disease or a clinical problem and includes questions on the aetiology, pathology, diagnosis, differential diagnoses, complications, assessment, management and treatment. Each question must be read carefully and every word noted, as they will have been constructed very carefully.

Although the words 'discuss' and a few synonyms imply a certain vagueness, the response must be precise and directed. Having read the question, the answer plan is based on the clinical data required. These will usually correspond to the checklist used to revise each disease.

Diagnosis and differential diagnoses are based on only three sources of information: namely, the **history**, **examination** and **investigation**. If the diagnosis is given, it may require confirmation from the same three sources. Assessment means diagnosis (history, examination, investigation), but adds the dimension of **severity** of the problems encountered. Management is assessment plus treatment. Although the term may be used loosely, implying just treatment in some questions, it is worth writing a few sentences on confirmation of diagnosis and severity of the problem being treated. Treatment should not be restricted to surgery, as many other problems may require to be sorted out first.

Other disciplines that may be involved must be considered, such as nursing, physiotherapy, occupational therapy, and drugs, chemotherapeutic agents and radiotherapy. Radiological intervention forms a major part of treatment in many diseases.

The plan outlining the areas to be covered can be in the answer book or on scrap paper. The plan should take three to six minutes for most essays and allows concentrated thought around the topic. On completion, a line is drawn through it to imply to the examiner that there is more to come, and the first few sentences of the introduction are constructed. This should imply an understanding of the topic, giving the examiner confidence that the essay is on the right track, and hopefully, is of good standard.

There is much debate as to whether headings should be underlined and key words highlighted. This debate is more of a problem to the candidate than the examiner, who is more concerned as to whether a script is legible, and demonstrates knowledge and understanding of the question. Illegibility is an inherent problem with some individuals. Examiners go to considerable effort to give candidates the benefit of the doubt but illegibility can never camouflage ignorance, and candidates would be well-advised to write at a rate at which the end product is guaranteed readable to the examiner.

Literacy and mastery of prose are more debatable. As much as examiners would wish medical graduates to be able to write skilfully and coherently, marks are predominantly awarded for factual knowledge and understanding of an essay topic. Success is, therefore, based on an appropriate plan and the development of each heading within it.

Medical schools and surgical colleges rarely set regular essays during their courses, even when they use this means of final assessment. It is, therefore, appropriate for students who know they will be examined in this way to undertake preliminary practice. A series of essay questions has, therefore, been added after the SAQ sections in each chapter. There is a section on planned structural outlines as a preliminary to writing essays and examples of good and poor answers with examiner's comments. These guidelines may be used to plan and write essays. The relevant practical information will usually be found in the sectional answers and teaching aids, and essays may be swapped with a working partner or discussion group, who would act as examiners. Subsequently, the plan, development, depth of knowledge, literary style and legibility is discussed. As the finals draw near, the pass standard becomes apparent, and essays can be accurately assessed by peer review.

Whichever examination system is chosen, it must be reliable, valid and discriminatory, and it should not be influenced by the subjective judgement of an examiner. The examination should be about the contents of a paper and not expertise or prior coaching in the chosen system. Nevertheless, it is essential to have prior exposure to the local examination system and be well-versed in its technique. This text is intended to provide that exposure and to educate candidates in the techniques of SAQ and essay writing in the hope of easing their passage to qualification.

APPENDIX B: SELF-ASSESSMENT SAQ PAPERS

Notes for Readers – SAQ Exam Papers

There are 12 questions in each paper, to be answered in two hours.

- You are advised to spend no more than 10 minutes on each question.
- The questions are designed to promote succinct answers.
- The marks awarded for each section are indicated.

Paper 1: 1.4, 2.1, 3.5, 3.6, 4.4, 5.5, 6.1, 7.2, 8.2, 9.4, 10.4, 11.1

Paper 2: 1.5, 2.2, 2.14, 3.7, 4.5, 5.6, 6.7, 7.3, 8.3, 9.5, 10.5, 11.2

Paper 3: 1.1, 2.11, 3.2, 3.8, 5.2, 5.7, 6.14, 7.4, 8.4, 9.10, 10.6, 11.3

Paper 4: 1.6, 2.4, 3.9, 4.7, 5.8, 6.8, 7.5, 8.5, 9.7, 10.7, 10.14, 11.5

Paper 5: 1.7, 2.16, 3.15, 4.8, 5.9, 6.3, 6.12, 7.11, 8.6, 9.8, 10.9, 11.6

Paper 6: 1.8, 2.6, 3.11, 4.9, 5.10, 6.6, 6.9, 7.8, 8.7, 9.9, 10.10, 11.7

Paper 7: 1.9, 2.7, 2.13, 3.4, 3.16, 5.11, 6.10, 7.7, 7.9, 8.8, 10.11, 11.8

Paper 8: 1.2, 2.5, 3.10, 4.6, 5.12, 6.2, 7.10, 7.12, 8.9, 9.2, 10.12, 11.9

Paper 9: 1.10, 2.8, 2.10, 3.12, 4.2, 5.4, 6.4, 7.13, 9.6, 9.12, 10.8, 10.13

Paper 10: 2.3, 2.15, 3.1, 4.10, 5.1, 6.11, 7.1, 8.1, 9.1, 10.1, 10.2, 11.11

Paper 11: 1.3, 2.9, 2.12, 3.3, 5.3, 6.5, 6.13, 7.6, 9.3, 10.3, 11.4, 10.13

APPENDIX C: SELF-ASSESSMENT ESSAY QUESTION PAPERS

Notes for Readers – Essay Exam Questions

There are four questions in each paper, to be answered in two hours.

- You are advised to spend no more than 30 minutes on each question and to spend the first five minutes formulating an outline for your answer.

Paper 1: 2.1, 4.1, 6.1, 8.1

Paper 2: 1.2, 2.2, 9.2, 11.2

Paper 3: 1.2, 2.3, 6.3, 10.3

Paper 4: 2.4, 5.4, 9.4, 11.4

Paper 5: 2.5, 5.5, 6.2, 8.2

Paper 6: 1.4, 3.1, 7.1, 10.5

Paper 7: 3.2, 5.3, 7.2, 11.1

Paper 8: 3.3, 4.2, 7.3, 8.3

Paper 9: 3.4, 6.4, 7.4, 10.4

Paper 10: 4.3, 9.3, 10.2, 11.3

Paper 11: 3.5, 5.1, 6.5, 7.7

Paper 12: 1.1, 5.2, 9.1, 10.1

ORDER FORM

Please send me:

- ☐ One copy of **OSCEs: Volume 1** £16.95
- ☐ One copy of **OSCEs: Volume 2** £16.95
- ☐ One copy of **Surgical Finals: Passing the Clinical** £13.95
- ☐ One copy of **Medical Finals: Passing the Clinical** £13.95
- ☐ One copy of **Medical Finals: SAQs and Essays** £13.95
- ☐ One copy of **150 Essential MCQs for Medical Finals** £11.95
- ☐ One copy of **150 Essential MCQs for Surgical Finals** £11.95

Free Postage on Books for Medical Students to UK Addresses

Name: ....

Address: ....

....

....

Daytime telephone number: ....

☐ I enclose a cheque/money order payable in sterling to PasTest Ltd. Please write your cheque guarantee card number and expiry date clearly on the back of your cheque

☐ Please debit my Access/Visa/Switch card

Card number: ....

Expiry date: .... Switch Issue Number: ....

Signature: ....

PasTest, FREEPOST,
Knutsford, Cheshire WA16 7BR, UK
Freephone 0800 980 0814

E-mail: books@pastest.co.uk
Website:http:// www.pastest.co.uk

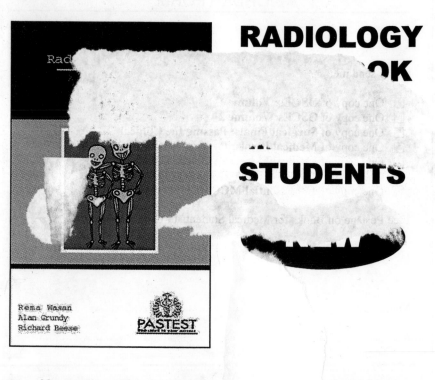